*Female Fertility and the
Body Fat Connection*

Women in Culture and Society

A SERIES EDITED BY CATHARINE R. STIMPSON

ROSE E. FRISCH

Female Fertility and the Body Fat Connection

WITH A FOREWORD BY ROBERT L. BARBIERI, M.D.

The University of Chicago Press • *Chicago and London*

Rose E. Frisch is associate professor of population sciences emerita at the Harvard School of Public Health and a member of the research faculty of the Harvard Center for Population and Development Studies. She is a fellow of the American Academy of Arts and Sciences and the John Simon Memorial Guggenheim Foundation. She is the editor of *Adipose Tissue and Reproduction* (1990) and has written widely on female fertility and on the natural fertility of populations.

The University of Chicago Press, Chicago 60637
The University of Chicago Press, Ltd., London
© 2002 by The University of Chicago
All rights reserved. Published 2002
Printed in the United States of America
11 10 09 08 07 06 05 04 03 02   1 2 3 4 5

ISBN: 0-226-26545-5 (cloth)

Library of Congress Cataloging-in-Publication Data

Frisch, Rose E. (Rose Epstein)
    Female fertility and the body fat connection / Rose E. Frisch.
        p.   cm.—(Women in culture and society)
    Includes bibliographical references and index.
    ISBN 0-226-26545-5 (cloth : alk paper)
    1. Fertility, Human.   2. Infertility, Female.   3. Body composition.   4. Human reproduction.   I. Title.
    II. Series.

RG136 .F755 2002
618.1′78—dc21

                                    2001053859

For
DAVID, HENRY, AND RUTH

and my parents,
LOUIS AND STELLA

CONTENTS

FOREWORD

The overarching goal of science is to discover unifying theories that explain the complex events that comprise our world. In physics, the study of the interaction of matter and energy has yielded a relatively few elegant and simple theories to explain our everyday experience of the motion of objects, sound and sight. In contrast to physics, the biological and social sciences are characterized by hundreds of complex theories that often have modest predictive value for explaining the events in our world. In *Female Fertility and the Body Fat Connection* Dr. Rose Frisch provides a thorough account of one of the most simple and elegant theories in biology: *in women, body fat provides the overarching control of the organs responsible for reproduction.* The text is both a personal and scholarly accounting of the discovery and proof of concept. Resonating with the elegance and simplicity of the theory, the text is straightforward and filled with layers of complexity.

A powerful and simple theory can help us understand ourselves, our neighbors, and the world at large. The idea that in women, food, working through body fat, can control sex and fertility can help answer questions such as, What determines the age of onset of menstruation? How does physical activity modulate the impact of food on sex and fertility? How does the relation between body fat and reproduction help to explain the physical changes that can be experienced by talented lean athletes such as ballet dancers, runners, and swimmers? How does the body fat–fertility connection help to explain the cause of infertility in some lean women? How does the body fat–fertility connection help to explain the reproductive potential of populations of women in countries with unique nutritional situations and habits? And finally,

How can you determine the range of weight which will help you achieve optimal health?

This book will be immensely helpful to women who want to know the connection between diet, exercise, and body fat with changes in their menstrual cycle, estrogen production, risk of infertility, and risk of disease such as breast cancer and osteoporosis. The body fat connection is a major determinant of our individual health and the health of the women in our country.

—Robert L. Barbieri, M.D.
Kate Macy Ladd Professor of Obstetrics, Gynecology, and Reproductive Biology, Harvard Medical School; chairman of the Department of Obstetrics and Gynecology and Reproductive Biology, Brigham and Women's Hospital, Boston

ACKNOWLEDGMENTS

I thank my collaborators and coauthors for their invaluable contributions during the three decades of research on "the body fat connection."

I am grateful to Drs. Seymour Reichlin, Freddy Homburger, Douglas Wilmore, and Roy Greep for their interest and encouragement in the early years of my research.

I am also grateful to the John Simon Guggenheim Memorial Foundation for the fellowship to study the biological determinants of female fecundity in 1975–76. A grant from the Population Council also supported this research. I thank R. J. Wolfe, the former Rare Books librarian at the Francis A. Countway Library of Medicine, Harvard Medical School, for his generous assistance with the historical medical data on this topic.

The research on the reproductive ability of the runners and swimmers at Harvard University and the Alumnae Health Study was conducted under the auspices of the Advanced Medical Research Foundation, Boston. Drs. Tenley Albright and Nile Albright of that Foundation were collaborators on the projects.

The research on the quantification of body fat by magnetic resonance imaging was supported by a grant from the National Institute of Child Health and Human Development, National Institutes of Health. I thank especially Drs. Robert Barbieri, chairman of the Department of Obstetrics and Gynecology, Brigham and Women's Hospital, Boston, and Bruce Rosen, director of the Nuclear Magnetic Resonance (NMR) Imaging Center, Massachusetts General Hospital, Boston, for their collaboration on the MRI research.

I thank Dr. Grace Wyshak, associate professor of biostatistics and population and international health, Harvard School of Public Health, for her collaboration and major contribution to the collection, analysis, and publication of the data of the Alumnae Health Study, still ongoing.

I thank Drs. Joel Cohen, Rudolph Leibel, and Janet W. McArthur for reading relevant chapters and for their comments.

I thank Susan Pedreira for the transcription of the manuscript, and Christopher Cahill and Helen Schmierer for their assistance. I thank Anthony Burton for his assistance with my queries.

I am grateful to my late husband, David Henry Frisch, a physicist who was a patient, often surprised, listener to the details of the research for many years.

I thank Michael Brehm for his cover design. I also thank editor Susan Bielstein for her perceptive advice. Finally, I am grateful to production editor Leslie Keros for her editorial assistance, insight, and support.

1 Female Body Fat

Celebrating the Difference

Since the dawn of human history, the symbols of female fertility have been fat, very fat—particularly in the places where the female sex hormone, estrogen, stores fat. Figure 1 below shows a typical fertility goddess, the Venus of Willendorf, dating from 30,000 B.C.; fortunately, she is only 4⅜ inches high. African, Asian, and Indian fertility goddesses in past centuries were also archetypal curvaceous females, a far cry from our current cult of the pencil-slim woman.

Why did the ancients have fertility goddesses? We can deduce that fertility was not an easy thing to achieve in the early times of our species because food was often in short supply. This ancient recognition of the connection between fatness and fertility proved to be a sound strategy for the maintenance of the species.

During the centuries up to our own times, artists have celebrated female body fat, but with considerably more restraint, as the Venus de Milo and the lush ladies in Peter Paul Rubens's paintings—two examples of many—illustrate. The historical linking of fatness and fertility makes sense to me biologically because, more than two decades ago, I discovered that women need a certain amount of fat to become fertile and remain fertile. I found that a girl does not have her first menstrual cycle (menarche) until she has a predictable minimum amount of body fat, and that a grown woman requires

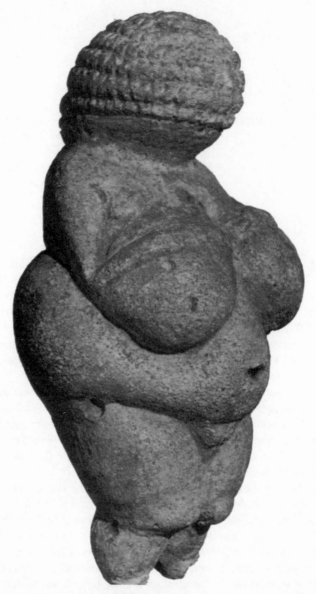

Figure 1. The Venus of Willendorf, a fertility figure, dating from 30,000 B.C. (fortunately, she is only 4⅜ inches high). She is fat in all the areas in which the hormone estrogen deposits fat. At present, she resides in the Natural History Museum in Vienna.

a larger minimum amount of fat to maintain ovulation and regular menstrual cycles.

SHE AND HE: DIVERSE BODIES

When I began researching why differing amounts of body fat could apparently turn menstrual cycles on or off, I had the entire field to myself. Body fat was not high on the agenda of reproductive endocrinologists. I began by reading everything I could find about body fat and the differences between the body fat of women and men.

Women at all ages have more body fat than men. It is at puberty, however, that the female attributes of rounded breasts, hips, buttocks, and thighs develop. Estrogen, the female hormone, begins to rise at this time, eventually reaching adult levels. Males, in contrast, become leaner as they become sexually mature at puberty.

The differing amounts of female and male fat are also distributed differently, as is normally very easy to observe. Men have more fat on the trunk and above the umbilicus (belly button). When men get fatter as they get older (which they do, just as women do, unless they work at avoiding it), that's where most of the new fat is added. Another male characteristic, not as well known, is the fat at the nape of the neck: it is thicker in men. In fact, this is the only area where fat is known to be thicker in men than in middle-aged women (that is, women about 40 years old). As women become fatter with age, they add fat below the umbilicus rather than above. Women may also have an increase of fat on the trunk after menopause.

A woman's body and a man's body differ internally as well as externally, a very important but not commonly observed fact. "Man," the medical textbooks state, is 60 percent water. Woman, as most textbooks neglect to state, is 50 percent water. And thereby hangs a tale. A 10 percent difference in body water may not seem significant, but it is. Fat contains very little water (5 to 10 percent), while muscles and internal organs contain a great deal of water (about 80 percent). The

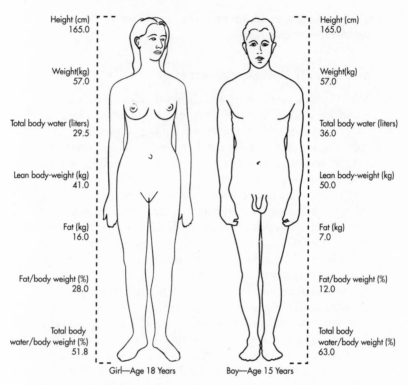

Figure 2. Comparison of the body composition of an 18-year-old girl and a 15-year-old boy of the same height and weight. Note the difference in the total body water/ body weight percentage, an index of fatness. Data from R. E. Frisch, "What's Below the Surface?" *New England Journal of Medicine* 305 (1981): 1019–20 (correspondence).

10 percent difference in body water translates into a much larger difference in body fat: in men body fat is 12 to 14 percent of body weight, and in women body fat is 26 to 28 percent of body weight.

The difference in body composition of a young woman and a young man of the same height and weight is shown in figure 2. The numbers are astonishing. By the time girls finish their growth in height and weight at about age 16 to 18, they have stashed away about 35 pounds (16 kg), 28 percent of their body weight, as fat: 144,000 calories. Boys complete their height and weight growth later than girls, at about age 18 to 20, and by that time they have stored only about 15 pounds (7 kg), 12 percent of their body weight, as fat: 63,000 calories. This large difference in body composition may be one of the most important differences characterizing women and men, because, as I found, all of that fat in women is related to their reproductive ability.

When I first calculated that a nonoverweight young woman had 35 pounds of fat in her body, I didn't believe it. Where is it all? I looked for direct dissection measurements in autopsy reports; there weren't many that recorded fat content, but the few that did confirmed the large amount of fat in adult women. Much of the fat is inside the abdomen, surrounding the internal organs. I asked my research assistant who had dissected a female corpse about it. "I removed the fat in buckets," she assured me. As women age, the proportion of body weight that is fat rises to 30 or 40 percent if they are well nourished. As men age, they also gain rapidly, until fat is 20 percent or even 30 percent of body weight.

Body Fat, an Active Metabolic Tissue

When researchers discovered the hormones controlling human reproduction about seventy years ago, body fat was considered to be an inert storage layer that insulated the body surface and acted as a protective cushion for delicate organs like the kidneys. The large difference in the relative fatness of women and men was not regarded as a potential determinant of or contributor to reproductive ability or sexuality any more than an electric blanket would have been.

In about 1940, however, researchers showed that body fat, or adipose tissue (the medical term, from the Latin *adeps,* "fat"), is metabolically active. Body fat actively participates in the maintenance of the body's energy balance; body fat cells (adipocytes) store fat as a potential source of energy and mobilize the fat into a fuel molecule when needed. Body fat, as I learned, is an amazing tissue, aside from its connection to fertility. Here are some basic facts.

To be of use to the body, the energy must be easily accessible for withdrawals or deposits. Although fat looks white or pale yellow in both humans and animals, it has a network of capillaries (small blood vessels) equal to that of muscle, so interactions with the circulatory system for the deposit and withdrawal of energy are efficient. Each fat cell has a connection to the sympathetic nervous system (the system of nerves that carries messages to the blood vessels and organs). The adrenal gland, a small gland located on top of each kidney, secretes a hormone that controls the flux of energy from the fat cells. Insulin, a hormone secreted in the pancreas, is the overall regulator of the input and outflow of free fatty acids from the fat cells that are used as energy, in addition to the sympathetic adrenal regulation.

Free fatty acids continually leave the fat cells as energy-rich materials to be used as fuel, or *oxidized,* by the heart, muscles, and the other organs of the body. The brain, however, can use only glucose, a carbohydrate, as a source of energy. During times of hunger, muscular activity, cold, or acclimation to cold, the flow of energy from the fat cells increases. After starvation and refeeding, fat cells accumulate fat. They can also accumulate fat after normal feeding.

Carbohydrates (starches and sugars) in the diet are converted into fat by the fat cells. How much of the glucose is stored as fat is regulated by your nutritional state: When not much carbohydrate is present, the conversion to fat is reduced; when a lot of carbohydrate is available, the storage is accelerated. In the steady state, about a third of the carbohydrate you eat is temporarily converted to fat.

WHY WE STORE ENERGY AS FAT

Why do we have this elaborate system for storing energy as fat? Why not store carbohydrates directly? There are very good reasons. If you stored energy as carbohydrates, you might not be able to move very quickly, and in prehistoric times your predators would have caught you. Calories from fat are stored directly in the fat cells without any conversion. In contrast, carbohydrate (glucose) is stored as glycogen in the liver and muscle, which requires the addition of water (which is heavy) and other substances. Fat stores energy more efficiently both because it does not require additional water and because it has a greater caloric density per gram (9 kilocalories) compared to carbohydrate (4 kilocalories).

A "THRIFTY" GENOTYPE

Centuries ago, in populations with marginal and fluctuating food supplies and a low caloric intake, women and men who stored energy as fat had a better chance of surviving when food supplies were low. They developed a "thrifty" genotype, which allowed them to store calories easily. But this ability, once an asset, has become a liability; today it means the easy accumulation of fat. The Pima Indians, for example, inherited this genotype, and as a result they have developed a high incidence of obesity and of diabetes associated with obesity. In the past, Pima Indians ate a low-fat, high-fiber diet of corn, beans, and indigenous plants, so obesity was not a problem. With a modern, high-fat diet, however, there is too high of an energy intake, and the energy is stored too easily.

BODY FAT AND ESTROGEN, THE FEMALE HORMONE

One of the surprising scientific discoveries of the twentieth century was that body fat converts androgens, the male hormone, to estrogens, the female hormone, by means of an enzyme called aromatase. With the help of this enzyme, which is found in the endoplasmic reticulum (intercellular mechanism) of the fat cells, the weak androgen, androstenedione, made mainly by the adrenal cortex (the outside layer of the adrenal gland), is converted to an estrogen.

By this process, called aromatization, all the estrogen produced by a woman after menopause comes from her body fat. About a third of the circulating estrogen of a premenopausal woman comes from aromatization of androgens to estrogen by her body fat.

If young women or men become obese, this extra-ovarian source of estrogen may be directly involved in reproductive disorders that accompany obesity. Some women who suffer from polycystic ovary disease, which is often associated with obesity, have a chronic lack of menstrual cycles (amenorrhea). Men who are obese may have gynecomastia (enlargement of the breasts). Even in nonobese women, the production of estrogen by fat tissue in the breast may contribute to the risk of breast cancer.

REPRODUCTION COSTS CALORIES

Returning to the basic question: Why does a woman store so much fat? Summing the answer: Because human reproduction has a high metabolic cost. Over the past century, most women who grew up in developed countries were well nourished, so the high metabolic cost of human reproduction was not considered, much less known. Until about twenty years ago, the big problem for young women was how *not* to get pregnant. Worries of how to get pregnant became common only with increased numbers of women who were either too slim (underweight) or too lean (not necessarily underweight because muscles are heavy). What these women often lacked was sufficient energy stored for reproduction, that is, sufficient body fat.

A successful pregnancy costs about 50,000 calories over and above normal metabolic requirements, such as the calories needed to breathe, digest food, and keep warm. To understand why a woman of reproductive age must store body fat if food supplies are low or fluctuating, consider what determines the viability of a normal baby at birth. The baby's chances of survival depend on birth weight, which in turn is determined primarily by the mother's prepregnancy weight and, independently, by her weight gain during pregnancy.

Nursing, or *lactation,* to use the scientific term, costs about 500 to 1,000 calories a day. It's calorie expensive to make human milk, as is growing a baby. In prehistoric times, nursing was a necessary part of successful reproduction. If a mother (or a surrogate) could not nurse her baby, the baby did not survive; no other suitable food was available. So, energy had to be stored for nursing during the early months of the baby's life.

At a conference on the relationship between maternal nutrition and lack of ovulation while a woman is nursing, Dr. H. L. Vis, a pediatrician from Brussels, gave a vivid example of the energy drain of nursing. He recounted that in a mountainous area with low food supplies, a nursing woman had part of her skin dyed blue so that she would be recognized as nursing and not be required to perform manual labor. Breast milk from poorly nourished women, it is interesting to note, has the *same* nutritional quality for the infant as the milk from well-nourished women. In a poorly nourished woman, the necessary calories are taken from her body tissues.

In developing countries, lactating mothers with relatively restricted diets usually have birth intervals of two to three years without the use of contraceptives, especially if they are doing physical work. In developed countries, however, lactating women may have a birth interval as short as a year if they are not protected by contraception (see chapter 11 for details). One can speculate that the prehistoric females who continued to ovulate, even though they were underweight and undernourished, left no viable offspring or did not survive themselves. They therefore had no descendants and vanished in the dark past. Selection would have favored females who stopped ovulating until the food supply was restored. Then these women could store enough energy to deliver a viable baby, even if the food supply fluctuated during their pregnancy or nursing.

The "Go" or "No" Signal by the Brain (Hypothalamus)

How did it fit together—the high caloric cost of pregnancy, the storage of large amounts of body fat, and the control of ovulation by the brain? I proposed that the "right" amount of female body fat signals "go" to a portion of the brain known as the hypothalamus. Body fat stored during a girl's adolescent growth is a logical signal, because body fat provides the energy needed for a successful pregnancy and for breast-feeding the infant in the months of rapid brain development after birth. Body fat also contributes to the estrogen levels necessary for ovulation. If this was true, then the reverse would also be true: if there is not enough body fat because of dieting or intensive physical activity, there is no ovulation, no menstrual cycle, and no pregnancy. Gain of body fat, then, would reverse the infertility.

About fifty years ago, Geoffrey Harris of Cambridge University discovered that the hypothalamus controls the ability to reproduce in addition to controlling food and water intake, body temperature, and emotions. He showed that the hypothalamus triggers the cascade of hormones that control the reproductive system. There seemed to be some feedback from the body to the brain, in effect reporting, "Yes, this body is 'grown up'; reproduction will be successful. Go ahead." What was the message?

Everybody knows that people "grow up" before becoming sexually mature. But how do you measure being grown up? "It's a matter of age, of course," you might answer. But chronological age by itself is not always a sufficient measure. Suppose a girl has been dieting or running thirty miles a week. She can be 16 years old and perfectly healthy, but, as I found, she still will not have had menarche, the first menstrual cycle. Some factor other than age must control sexual maturation.

You can see why age could be a disastrous criterion for sexual maturation in poor countries devastated by food shortages. There, the body weight of a 16-year-old girl can be as low as that of a 9-year-old girl in a well-fed population. It wouldn't be good for the girl—or the species—if sexual maturation were determined by age alone. She would not be able to reproduce successfully.

Height does not define sexual maturation, either; early-maturing girls tend to have menarche at a shorter height than do late-maturing girls (though both share the same average height when they complete their growth at age 18).

What about body weight? Body weight, I found, did make a difference, particularly the weight gained by girls during their rapid adolescent growth, which always occurs before the first menstrual cycle. But body weight includes so many organs and tissues; what was the important component of body weight? As the reader now knows, the critical factor turned out to be the amount of body fat in relation to the amounts of muscle and bone in a girl or woman.

My first published report on fatness and fertility, co-authored with Dr. J. W. McArthur, then a gynecologist at Massachusetts General Hospital, was titled explicitly: "Menstrual Cycles: Fatness as a Determinant of Minimum Weight for Height Necessary for their Maintenance or Onset." Published in *Science* in 1974, it created quite a stir. "How could fatness matter?" was a typical reaction. But clinicians began using the reported minimum weights designated by our "fatness index" (described in chapter 6), and they succeeded in restoring fertility when its loss was caused by excessive thinness. I was cheered when the late Karl Cori, a Nobel laureate biochemist, told me he had read my paper in *Science* and had said, "*There's* something new."

"Moderate" Weight Loss and Suppression of Cycles

It still astonishes some women—and most men—that menstrual cycles can either stop or not start at all if a woman or girl of normal weight loses even 10 or 20 pounds. For example, if a woman is five feet five inches tall, her normal weight is about 125 pounds, so losing 10 to 20 pounds represents about 10 to 15 percent of the normal weight for her height. Weight loss in that range is mainly loss of fat (in fact, it is a loss of about one-third of the total storage of body fat). When I began my research, fat loss in that range was not considered a possible reason for the absence or delay of menstrual cycles. Anorectic girls do not menstruate, but they lose about 30 percent of the normal weight for their height; they lose both fat and muscle mass.

Doctors, and everyone else, were even more surprised when my fellow researchers and I reported that ballet dancers, and then women runners, swimmers, and rowers, had irregular menstrual cycles or no cycles when they engaged regularly in intensive exercise. The athletes and dancers also were surprised, and often upset, by the lack of cycles. "Stress" was the reason given by almost everyone but me.

When I brought up the subject, which I often did because I was totally immersed in the research, people typically responded with, "You mean those young women are infertile? What about those gymnasts who look so little?"

"Yes, they are infertile," I would reply. "They do not have any menstrual cycles, or menarche is very delayed; gymnasts are a good example of the delay." If nonmedical men asked the question, they reacted with general consternation and shock to the phrase "menstrual cycles." Even "menarche" sounded dangerously taboo, although most adults no longer know what menarche means (*mens,* "month"; *arche,* "beginning"). Once, when I gave a talk to an assembly of distinguished economists on this topic, they seemed to think at first that menarche was a new kind of vegetable.

Any Body Will Not Do

How I arrived at the unexpected significance of body composition is the subject of the next chapter. But here is a question animal breeders ask that sets the stage: *What do we want in a carcass?* For humans, translate "carcass" as "the body."

In 1974 I had the good fortune to attend a NATO symposium titled "Meat Animals" at the invitation of David Lister, then of the Bristol Meat Research Institute in England. Dr. Lister was a former student of Robert McCance, a Cambridge University professor and distinguished researcher on the body composition of mammals. I had sent Dr. McCance a hypothetical scheme of how and why I thought a critical amount of body fat was necessary for sexual maturation. Dr. McCance wrote me that he thought my hypothesis "wrapped things up well," and he was going to speak about it at the Royal Society in London, of which he was a member. "If he's going to speak about it, I will be there," I told my husband, and took off for London. At that meeting I met Dr. Lister, who was having difficulty breeding pigs because the public wanted very lean pork and that meant breeding very lean pigs. But the very lean pigs were relatively infertile—they had very few piglets. So, Dr. Lister, who had already heard of my ideas on fertility and body fat, invited me to attend the NATO conference.

At the symposium I learned from animal breeders about the changes in muscle, bone, and body fat of pigs, cattle, and sheep as the animals mature sexually. How quickly or slowly these changes take place in different breeds of domestic animals is important economically for both animal breeding and meat production. Therefore, these components of body composition are studied extensively in England. Carcasses are dissected into pieces weighing only a few grams (one gram equals 0.035 ounces) at various stages of growth to determine the exact proportions of muscle and fat. Marbling fat in beef, I learned, develops last; it is sex fat. Veal is low in fat because it is from sexually immature calves.

These basic and illuminating facts are reported in *Farm Animals,* a book by Cambridge University researcher Sir John Hammond. Looking for the equivalent data for women and men, I found it in a volume at Harvard's Countway Library of Medicine: *The Body Cell Mass,* by Dr. Francis D. Moore and his large group of collaborators. When the book was written, Dr. Moore was chief of surgery at Brigham and Women's Hospital in Boston and a pioneer in the study of human body composition. These two books provided the groundwork for my early research linking fat and fertility.

The question animal breeders ask, "What do we want in a carcass?" seems very crude. But it was the right question to ask, to put the body back in the human reproductive picture. As I found, any body will not do (pun intended).

2   Too Little and Too Much Body Fat

"Tell me what you eat, and I will tell you what you are," said Jean A. Brillat-Savarin, the nineteenth-century French physiologist and lawyer, in his celebrated book *The Physiology of Taste*. After more than twenty years of research connecting fatness and fertility, I propose a new version of the old aphorism: Tell me what *and how much* you eat, *and tell me how many miles a day you run or jog or hours you dance,* and I'll tell you *how fertile* you are.

For three decades I studied women who had too little body fat—they dieted too much or exercised too much or both. These girls and women were not anorectics. Anorexia nervosa is a well-known psychogenic disease, one that originates in the mind. Anorectic girls starve themselves and lose one-third or more of their body weight—fat and lean body weight. The super slim, super lean women in my studies represented a new phenomenon: they ate, but only enough to be slim and lean. Their diet consisted mostly of nonfat yogurt, lettuce, pasta, and gallons of diet drinks.

A "TURNED-OFF" REPRODUCTIVE SYSTEM

In the mid-1970s, a surprisingly large number of these super slim, super lean women called me at Harvard's Center for Population Studies, part of the Harvard School of Public

Health, where I was a professor of population sciences. They were experiencing an assortment of reproductive problems, and they contacted me after reading about my research on body fat and fertility in a magazine or newspaper. Their periods had stopped or become very irregular or had never started at all. Or they wanted to have a child but they hadn't been able to become pregnant.

By the time they contacted me, these super slim, super lean women already had been to a doctor for a complete physical. (I always checked that they had seen their doctor since it is important to rule out other possible causes of infertility.) "My doctor told me there's nothing wrong physically with my reproductive system," they said. "It just seems to be 'turned off.'" Sometimes they reported that their doctor had said that "it could be stress." More recently, having learned of my research, their doctor had told them that they may be "too thin."

I vividly remember a call from one young woman who told me in a whisper, "I don't have any . . ." Her voice dropped so low that I couldn't hear what she didn't have, though I could guess. Joan, as I will call her, taught second grade in an elementary school in a small southern town. The only phone she could use during the workday was in the main hallway of the school, with schoolchildren running around her. So she whispered that she and her husband wanted a child but that she had no menstrual cycles. You can understand why she didn't tell me this in loud, ringing tones.

Joan went on to tell me that she ran "just" thirty-five miles a week and ate a low-calorie, nonfat diet. Her doctor had found nothing wrong with her reproductive system, and Joan desperately wanted to know what she should do so that she could become pregnant.

I inquired about her height and weight. When she told me that she was five foot five inches tall and weighed 103 pounds, I was certain that I understood the reason for her problem. Her weight was far below the normal, average weight of 125 pounds for her height. She needed to gain weight—at least five to eight pounds—to be above the minimum weight for her height for the occurrence of ovulation and menstrual cycles. I told her she could do two things: cut back on her running and increase her caloric intake. She could add some calories from fat to her diet by drinking 1 percent milk instead of skim and by eating low-fat yogurt instead of nonfat.

Joan's story has a happy ending. She gained weight and became pregnant, as she told me in another whispered phone call several months later. About a year after her first call, I received in the mail a photograph of her smiling baby daughter.

Other women who have called me hoping to have a baby have not experienced such a happy ending. Take Ellen, a forty-year-old champion athlete who had worn nothing larger than a size two for twenty years. Newly married, she and her husband very much wanted to have a child. Following my suggestion that she try to gain weight to restore ovulation and her menstrual cycles, Ellen ate toast with cream cheese every morning and consumed quarts of ice cream. Her husband, she reported, was delighted when her breasts began to enlarge. But though she attended an excellent clinic for assisted reproduction, she did not succeed in conceiving. Fecundity begins to decline after about age 35, and by the time a woman reaches 40, her ability to conceive has decreased substantially. Even if she gains weight and reverses her excessive leanness, a woman over 35 can still fail to conceive. She needs to gain weight at a younger age.

STAGES OF TURNING OFF AND ON

As doctors have learned more about these super lean dieters and athletes, they have found that the disruption of reproductive ability is not an all-or-nothing process; the "turning off" occurs in stages. As a woman eats less or exercises more, the deleterious effect on her reproductive system increases. Doctors call this relationship a dose response.

A woman might have what appears to be a normal menstrual cycle, but when she tries to become pregnant, she does not succeed. That is because, although her cycle appears to be normal, ovulation—the release of an egg from the ovary—is not occurring. If she becomes thinner or leaner, her menstrual cycles may become irregular and infrequent and then stop completely. That is when too thin or too lean women go to see a doctor.

A girl who trains intensively before menarche (the first cycle) may not have her first menstrual cycle until as late as age 19 or 20. Mothers of such girls become frantic, worrying that their athletic daughters are abnormal. (They are not.) Menarche is achieved with weight gain or reduction of activity or both.

If everything else is normal, women with amenorrhea (absence of cycles) can reverse these disruptions of reproductive ability by gaining weight or decreasing athletic activity or both. The time it takes to resume normal, regular cycles usually depends on how long the cycles have been turned off. The longer they have been turned off, the longer it takes for them to turn on.

Like the response to weight loss, the response to weight gain occurs in stages. As a woman's weight enters the normal range, regular menstrual cycles may resume without ovulation at first. Then, as the woman gains more weight, normal ovulation also resumes.

If a woman who is too lean because of intense athletic training cuts back on her athletic activity, she will start normal, regular cycles again even if her weight remains the same. This occurs because the proportion of muscle and fat—the body composition—changes even though the weight is stable. If less of the woman's weight is muscle and more is fat, the proportion necessary to maintain regular cycles is attained.

Amazingly, a weight change of as little as three to five pounds above or below the threshold weight can be enough to turn the cycle on or off. Apparently, the hypothalamus, the part of the brain that controls reproduction, responds to a very small difference in relative fatness in an adult woman. One of the swimmers we studied was a clear example of this.

My collaborators and I recorded the menstrual histories of undergraduate athletes in a yearlong study of the effects of exercise on the menstrual cycle. Each athlete reported regularly on her cycle as the study proceeded, so we knew who had cycles and who did not. One of our expert swimmers, a Harvard undergraduate, suddenly reported a normal four-day period. Her record showed that she had not had a period in five months, so I was surprised. I called her and asked if she had done anything different in the past month.

"Oh, yes," she said. "I gained five pounds."

"How?" I asked.

"I packed carbohydrates for a month," she replied.

"Why?" I asked.

"I was curious to see if there was anything to your hypothesis," she said.

This swimmer was five feet seven inches tall and had weighed 108 pounds, which I could predict was about four pounds below the minimum critical weight—112 pounds for her height—for the occurrence of regular menstrual cycles.

"Are you going to keep on having menstrual cycles?" I asked.

"Oh, no," she replied. "I'll lose the five pounds next month." She did, and she had no more cycles.

Some gymnasts told me that they turned cycles on and off with a three-pound weight change around the critical weight for their height. Usually, however, only the minimum weight for height at which cycles are possible can be predicted, not the weight above the minimum at which cycles actually resume. I will discuss minimum weights further in chapter 6.

INFERTILITY WITH OBESITY AND "YO-YOING"

What about too much fat? Very obese women are also infertile. So are "overfed heifers, sheep, pigs and mares," as a great English physiologist, Francis Marshall, reported more than a century ago. Marshall described an infertile hackney mare who was purposely kept very fat for the comfort of her rider, an elderly and presumably very nervous gentleman. "When much reduced," Marshall observed, the mare became fertile again. Starvation restores the fertility of overfed animals, and weight loss restores the fertility of excessively fat women. We are not yet sure what the mechanisms are that cause the infertility attributed to excessive fatness; it is still a relatively new phenomenon in the history of our species to have so much food that we can become too fat.

If a woman's weight fluctuates up and down, or yo-yos, in the range where she is losing and gaining fat, her brain will also turn off her reproductive ability. To reproduce, the body apparently needs to maintain a steady supply of stored energy. It is as if the hypothalamus can't figure out who you are when your body composition fluctuates wildly: are you grown up enough to reproduce or are you still prepubertal? One of the early papers that I read reported on this yo-yoing effect among Japanese women, in addition to confirming the disruptive effect of having too little or too much fat.

"LEPTIN IS A GORGEOUS MOLECULE"

How does your brain know how fat or thin you are and then make the connection to your reproductive ability? One answer is leptin, a recently discovered hormone made by body fat that plays a key role in regulating food intake and energy metabolism. Leptin was identified in 1994 by researcher Jeffrey Friedman and his colleagues at Rockefeller University's Laboratory for Molecular Genetics; they cloned a gene that encoded leptin.

"Leptin is a gorgeous molecule," I was quoted as saying in a 1997 *New York Times* article about the discovery of leptin.[1] I do think leptin is a gorgeous, marvelous molecule, and not only because it provides the biochemical basis for my critical-fatness hypothesis. As I recount in detail later, leptin is made by all the fat cells in the body in both women and men; women, not surprisingly, have more leptin than men. Receptors for leptin are located in the hypothalamus, the part of the brain that controls food intake, energy metabolism, and reproductive ability. The story is still unfolding, and I discuss it further in chapters 3 and 10.

1. N. Angier, "Chemical Tied to Fat Control Could Help Trigger Puberty," *New York Times,* January 7, 1997, C1.

BROWN FAT

A special type of body fat that also makes leptin is *brown fat;* it is present in humans and hibernating mammals such as the groundhog and the opossum. Brown fat actually looks brownish red because it has a large number of heat-producing cellular particles called *mitochondria*. Brown fat makes heat; that is its purpose rather than storage of energy. Nobody knows whether brown fat is involved in reproduction.

At birth human babies have brown fat at the back of the neck, between the shoulder blades, around the groin, and under the armpits. Many other baby mammals have brown fat in the same places. Very young mammals cannot control their body temperature, and brown fat helps keep them warm.

Some researchers think that in human adults, some of the fat around the kidney and the thymus contains brown fat. If this is so, I theorize that by producing heat, brown fat increases the circulation rate of blood in these important organs without having to raise the metabolic rate of the whole body. This may explain why we don't have to eat continuously all day, the way the hummingbird does, to maintain a high metabolic rate.

FAT AND SEX IN MORE LOWLY CREATURES

The close connection between fatness and fertility is not unique to humans. Storage of lipid (fat) and the production of eggs and sperm are linked in such lowly, invertebrate creatures as starfish, oysters, and snails. Fat reserves, often stored in special organs, are used up during the time of reproduction. Fish such as salmon and herring store lipid reserves within and between muscles; these are relatively fatty fish, as you can tell by their taste. When salmon and herring reproduce, the fat and protein in the muscles are transferred to the gonads (ovaries or testes). In frogs, each gonad has an "adipose body" (fat body) spread between it and the kidney.

Even ants store fat for egg formation. Termite queens and kings have royal "adipose tissue"; how royal fat differs from plain old plebeian fat is not clear.[2] (Some insects use their adipose body for waste disposal. "The adipose body of old cockroaches is just one large mass of urates," a possibly useful piece of information you can stow away.)[3] Fortunately, our human adipose tissue stores only lipids.

Many birds also depend on stored fat for reproduction. Snow geese and other Arctic water birds build up fat during the spring migration and just before breeding. Among mammals, the development of fat under the skin (subcutaneous fat) varies with the degree of exposure to cold and the amount of fur the animal has. The fattest mammals, including whales, seals, pigs, and humans, have little body hair. Conversely, nonhuman primates such as monkeys and chimpanzees have little subcutaneous fat, presumably because of their large amount of hair. Cats, lions, and tigers, all carnivorous animals, also have little adipose tissue. Most of our domestic female animals, such as cattle, sheep, and pigs, experience an increase of fat at the time of sexual maturation, as does the human female. We can think of it as "sex fat," providing the energy for reproduction.

2. J. Vague and R. Fenasse, "Comparative Anatomy of Adipose Tissue," in *Adipose Tissue*, Handbook of Physiology, Section 5, ed. A. E. Renold and G. F. Cahill Jr. (Washington, D.C.: American Physiological Society, 1965), 27.

3. Ibid., 28.

3 · Female Adolescence
Puberty and Growing Up

You may never have heard of the adolescent "growth spurt"—a sudden, rapid growth first in height, then in weight—but if you are grown up, you have had it. A girl's growth spurt always occurs before menarche. In well-nourished populations like that of the United States, girls experience the spurt beginning at about age 9; boys experience it at about age 11.

Some researchers and the media use the word *puberty* to include all the physical changes that happen around and during the time of the growth spurt. Puberty is a rather fuzzy term that can denote the years of rapid adolescent growth, the appearance of secondary sex characteristics such as breast development and pubic hair, and menarche. Instead of using the category "puberty," I will refer separately to the adolescent growth spurt, the first "growing up" event that lasts for about three years; the development of secondary sex characteristics; and menarche, which follows the spurt.

Together with Roger Revelle (former director of the Harvard Center for Population Studies, where I conduct my research), I spent several years in the late 1960s and early 1970s learning about the weight changes that occur in girls during the adolescent growth spurt. (I'll tell you why shortly.) In that phase of the research, we made a new and important finding: menarche was closely related to a "critical" body weight. We were totally surprised at the connection to body weight. I soon found by reading about other species, however, that girls are just like other mammals, including monkeys and apes, in that sexual maturity is more closely related to body weight than to chronological age.

How did we ever come to research something so crude as kilograms of body weight? (A kilogram is equivalent to 2.2 pounds.) I was trained as a geneticist, and Roger was a well-known oceanographer; neither of us had been interested in body weights. We were inspired to look into adolescence and sexual maturation by our studies of body weight that had nothing to do with either topic—a good way to discover something new in science. At the time we were working on a Harvard project to calculate future world food needs. To estimate calorie requirements, you first have to know the body weights of the population you are planning to feed, so I collected body weight data for females and males of all ages, from birth to age 65 and older, from many developing countries.

An Unexpected Finding

Collecting all those body weights was somewhat boring, so I looked for the age of the largest yearly gain in weight of girls in various populations of developing countries. I knew that this "peak weight gain" always took place before menarche, and I was curious to know at just what age it took place. (Age of menarche was not reported.) For example, I found that Pakistani girls had their largest weight gain at age 13. I could infer, then, that menarche would occur for these girls sometime after that age, probably at 14 or 15.

But then something quite intriguing turned up. Within a generally undernourished population like Pakistan, poor rural girls experienced this peak weight gain at a later age (14) than did better-nourished urban girls (12). This finding agreed with previously published reports showing that poorly nourished girls had their growth spurt and menarche later than did well-nourished girls. What was unexpected was that the rural and urban girls had the *same average weight* at the time of the peak weight gain, although they peaked at different ages. Did the weight itself mean something? If so, what did it represent?

I decided to pursue this interesting discovery. I repaired to the library and began reading the literature on body size at all stages of a girl's sexual maturation. I found many research papers, but most of them focused on height rather than weight. When I inquired among anthropologists and pediatricians about the reason for the lack of detailed research on body weight, I was told that body weight was so variable that it was not worth studying in relation to sexual maturation. But as newcomers to the subject, neither Roger nor I had any such prejudice, so we did look at body weight.

ANALYZING GROWTH DATA: THE GIRLS' SPURT

To use the most accurate growth data, we relied on longitudinal growth studies in which the same girls were measured regularly as they grew up. In the studies we analyzed, the height and weight of each girl was measured every six months from birth to age 18, and her age of menarche was recorded. There were three such studies of girls and boys in the United States, one in Berkeley (California), one in Boston, and one in Denver. In all three, the subjects were well nourished and middle class.[1] The studies were completed in 1940–1950. We needed all three studies to get a large enough sample because there is always a great deal of variability in human growth.

1. It is important to compare persons of similar socioeconomic backgrounds, as studies have shown that age of growth and maturation differ by social class. See H. P. Bowditch, *Eighth Annual Report* (Boston: Massachusetts State Board of Health, 1877); V. Kiil, *Skrifter utgitt av det Norske Videnskaps-Akademi i Oslo* 2, no. 1 (1939). Kiil's data, collected from different social classes and geographic regions in Norway over 100 years, show "an undoubted connection between the age of the individual at the time sexual maturity commenced and the social conditions under which that person lives" (p. 145).

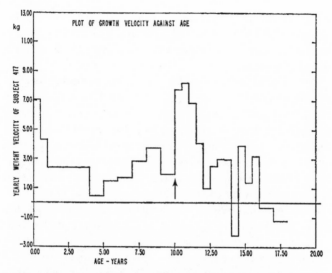

Figure 3. The amount of body weight gained each year (in the vertical axis, the weight gain is measured in kilograms; one kilogram equals 2.2 pounds), from birth to age 18, of one girl in the Denver study. The arrow shows the initiation of the adolescent growth spurt in weight at age 10. The rapid rise in weight gain is the spurt, which occurs before menarche, the first menstrual cycle. This girl, a rapid grower, had menarche at age 12.3. As the diagram shows, weight gain slows before menarche. From R. E. Frisch, "The Critical Weight at Menarche and the Initiation of the Adolescent Growth Spurt, and the Control of Puberty," in *Control of the Onset of Puberty*, ed. M. M. Grumbach, G. D. Grave, and F. E. Mayer (New York: John Wiley & Sons, 1974), 404. Copyright © 1974 by John Wiley & Sons, Inc. Reprinted with permission of John Wiley & Sons, Inc.

Figure 3 shows the annual weight gain of one of the girls from birth to age 18. (I plotted similar curves of height and weight gain for each of the 181 girls in the studies.) This girl was a rapid grower and an early maturer. The arrow in the diagram indicates when her growth spurt in weight began at age 10; that sudden, rapid rise in weight gain is "the spurt." The girl's fastest growth in weight occurred at age 12. As you can see in the diagram, menarche occurs after weight gain starts to slow down; in this girl, menarche occurred at 12 years and 4 months (12.3 years). The average age of menarche of the 181 girls was 12 years and 10 months (12.8 years).

What starts that rapid acceleration in growth before menarche? Researchers are still not sure of the control mechanisms, but two things are certain: every normal adolescent girl and boy has the growth spurt before maturing sexually, and adolescents starting the growth spurt eat, eat, and eat; it's hard to keep enough food in stock. Then, after the peak gain in weight, both weight gain and food intake decrease. Little is known about what controls the reduction in food intake. In fact, we still don't know why human beings have an adolescent growth spurt at all. Why not idle along at the same growth rate until menarche?

All mammals seem to have a growth spurt before sexual maturation, but we don't know why this happens, either. One possible reason for the growth spurt in humans is that the rapid growth for girls is accompanied by a large increase in stored, easily mobilized energy—body fat—useful for successful reproduction.

Timing of the "Spurt" and Menarche

In the studies we analyzed, girls began the adolescent growth spurt at 9.5 years of age on average. Menarche occurred about three years after the start of the spurt, at 12.8 years. Many teachers and parents are still surprised at these early ages. Girls experienced the fastest growth in height at 11.5 years of age on average, and their peak weight gain occurred about six months later, at age 12. However, there is a lot of variability around these average ages; this variability is measured statistically by the *standard deviation* (often abbreviated as SD).

In our study, the standard deviation of the ages for each of these adolescent events was about one year. For example, the average age of menarche was 12.8 years with a standard deviation of one year. This means that two-thirds of the girls had menarche between the ages of 11.8 (the average age, 12.8, minus one year) and 13.8 (the average age, plus one year).

Growth rates are so variable because how quickly or slowly you grow at all ages is controlled genetically; you inherit your growth rate. But growth rate can also be affected by environmental factors such as the quality and quantity of food you eat and the amount of energy you expend. Two girls in the same family who eat the same food and have the same environment can grow at very different rates, one fast and one slow. The genetically fast grower will mature sexually before the slow grower does. However, the fast grower will mature later if she diets to become super slim or if she runs twenty miles a week. And the slow grower will mature even later if she changes her life style similarly. Nutrition and energy outputs interact with the genetic control.

WEIGHT AT MENARCHE

Pediatricians conduct growth studies of healthy, normal children, like the studies I analyzed, to establish standards of height and weight for girls and boys at each age. Then they are able to assess whether a girl or boy is growing normally.

Oddly, even though the age of menarche was noted precisely for each of the girls in the growth studies we analyzed, apparently no one had ever asked the simple question, what is the height and weight of girls at menarche? After we determined the average height and weight, we especially wanted to know whether early and late menarcheal girls had the same weight at menarche. This was easy to find out because we had each girl's exact age of menarche and her height and weight at every age up to 18. It just took time to gather the data for 181 girls.

We were excited by the answers. For all the girls, the average weight at menarche was 103 pounds (47 kg), and the average age of menarche was 12 years and 10 months (12.8 years). And eureka! Similar to our earlier results on peak weight gain, the early- and late-maturing girls had the *same* average weight, 103 pounds (47 kg), whether they were younger than 12.8 years or older than 12.8 years at menarche. In 1970 Roger and I published this unexpected result in *Science* magazine, with some speculations as to what it could mean. The reaction to our article was usually incredulity: how could body weight matter? A good question that I set out to answer.

It was already known that height at menarche differed for early and late maturers. The average height for all girls at menarche was 62 inches (158 cm), but late-maturing girls were on average taller at menarche than the earlier maturers. I could now explain why many researchers reported that early maturers had more weight for height than did late maturers: average weights at menarche of early and late maturers are the same, but early maturers are shorter at menarche than late maturers.

When I reported these menarcheal height and weight results and their possible significance at a conference of pediatricians, I was greeted at first with dead silence. Then I was asked, "What is your background, Dr. Frisch?" (the tone of voice implying, how come are you here?). "I have my doctoral degree in genetics," I replied. "And who is Roger Revelle?" someone asked, mispronouncing "Revelle" to rhyme with "jelly." "Oh, Roger is an oceanographer," I answered, "and the director of the Population Center, where I work." More silence. No one apparently thought our new findings on weight at menarche mattered, and my presence was considered one of those aberrations that can happen at a conference. The response didn't trouble me. I had presented my message, and the doctors were polite.

I had been invited to speak at the conference by Dr. Thomas E. Cone Jr., then of Children's Hospital in Boston. Dr. Cone had read our published papers on the weight of girls and the adolescent spurt, including menarche. He was an expert on children's growth, and he found our results provocative and interesting. There were other doctors who also thought, as we did, that we were on to something, and they encouraged us to continue. But soon I learned that clinical doctors and researchers in any field, be it pediatrics, gynecology, or anthropology, are often uninterested in new ideas. Some scientists are even hostile to them, especially if the ideas come from a researcher they've never heard of who works in an unrelated discipline (like me). A famous biochemist at Harvard Medical School once asked me, perhaps overly pessimistically, "How do you think new ideas advance, Dr. Frisch?" "I'm not too sure," I replied, thinking of some of my recent experiences. "Funeral by funeral is the answer," he said.

Overall, I had an exciting time pursuing this research. I found that when I had good questions to ask, I could call or write experts in a field, and most would respond generously with answers and advice. In fact, that is how I met some of my co-investigators and mentors. I also followed the sage advice I read in a scientist's memoir (I can't remember whose): choose the experts in a field whom you respect most for knowledge and advice, and ignore the reactions of everybody else.

EARLIER MENARCHE: GIRLS "GROW UP" FASTER

Even before being able to predict menarche for an individual girl, I could explain the well-known but unexplained fact that menarche had occurred progressively earlier during the past one hundred years. As I found, historical studies showed that the average weight at menarche of girls in the United States was the same in the past as it is now, 103 pounds (47 kg). What happened about a century ago was that girls began to grow more quickly in both height and weight because of improved nutrition and a decrease in childhood disease. They became larger sooner and therefore reached the average weight at menarche at an earlier age.

As shown in figure 4 below, the average age of menarche in Europe has become earlier by two to three months per decade over the past century and a half. In the mid-1800s, for example, menarche occurred as late as age 17 in Scandinavia; one hundred years later, the average age had declined to

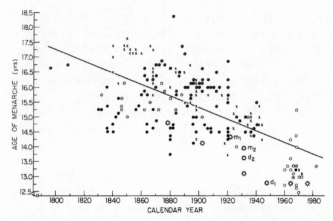

Figure 4. Mean (average) or median (middle of the distribution) age of menarche (years) as a function of calendar year from 1790 to 1980. The symbols refer to England (⊙); France (●); Germany (⊗); Holland (□); Scandinavia (Denmark, Finland, Norway, and Sweden) (×); Belgium, Czechoslovakia, Hungary, Italy, Poland (rural), Romania (urban and rural), Russia, Spain, and Switzerland (all labeled ○); and the United States (✲) (U.S. data not included in the regression line). The age of menarche has already leveled off in some European countries as it has in the United States (see U.S. data and text). Reprinted from G. Wyshak and R. E. Frisch, "Evidence for a Secular Trend in Age of Menarche," *New England Journal of Medicine* 306 (1982): 1033. Copyright © 1982 by the Massachusetts Medical Society. All rights reserved. Reprinted with permission of Grace Wyshak and the Massachusetts Medical Society.

about 14.5. In the United States, the average age of menarche was 14.7 in 1880 and declined to age 14 by 1900. Thereafter menarche occurred earlier by about three months per decade until 1945, when it leveled off at age 12.6 to 12.8.

Since the average age of menarche was 15.5 or 16 a century and a half ago, doctors then defined precocious puberty (abnormally early menarche) as menarche at age 11 or 12. Those ages are now close to the present average age of menarche, 12.6 to 12.8. Doctors now define precocious puberty as menarche at age 8 or 9.

I once heard an eminent anthropologist predict that menarche would become earlier and earlier, so eventually menarche might occur at age 6. First graders! What a thought! It cannot be so.

AGE OF MENARCHE NOW LEVELED OFF

Because menarche is a measure of how quickly girls grow, when girls' growth rates level off, the average age of menarche also levels off. As shown in the figure above, this is what has happened in the United States. Twelve-year-old girls have been the same average height and weight for more than fifty years. They have had good nutrition, and they no longer contract many of the childhood diseases that might slow their growth. Therefore, the average age of menarche has remained the same for the past fifty years as well.

Parents are apparently just becoming aware that the age of menarche is earlier now than it was a century ago. Puberty has become a popular subject in the media, and journalists often consult me to find out the facts. Confusion reigns about the timing of the "first menses," as one interviewer hesitantly described it. In summary, menarche is earlier today than in 1890 and 1900 for girls in the United States, but the trend to an earlier age of menarche has stabilized at 12.6 to 12.8 years.

FACTORS DELAYING THE AGE OF MENARCHE

Confirming the connection between the age of menarche and how rapidly or slowly girls grow in a particular population, any factor that slows weight growth before or after birth delays the age of menarche. Menarche occurs later in twins than in single-born children, for example, because twins grow more slowly. Malnutrition and undernutrition, both widespread among children in developing countries, delay menarche. Chronic childhood diseases in the United States, such as juvenile diabetes, sickle cell anemia, and cystic fibrosis, also slow growth and delay menarche. High altitude delays menarche by slowing the rate of weight growth both before and after birth; some of the latest average ages of menarche in the world, 17 and 18, occur in poorly nourished girls living at high altitudes in Peru and New Guinea. Then there are the athletes and dancers, who, as we found, fit the same model by undereating and overexercising, thus delaying menarche to the age of 15, 16, 17, or even 20.

A Mile High: Later Menarche of Denver Girls

Girls from Denver provide a particularly good example of how the natural environment can affect growth rate and thus the age of menarche. In the studies we analyzed, Denver girls were well nourished and middle class, as were the Berkeley and Boston girls. But Denver girls had menarche later, at an average age of 13, compared to 12.8 years for the two other groups. Although small, this difference was statistically significant. I couldn't figure out the reason for it until I read that at high altitudes growth in the uterus is slowed, resulting in lighter birth weights for both girls and boys.

But Denver is only a mile above sea level; would that be enough to affect birth weight? Indeed it is. When I added up the birth weights of the girls from Denver, they were 200 grams (7 oz) lighter on average than the birth weights of the girls in the sea-level cities of Berkeley and Boston. Birth weights of the boys from Denver averaged 400 grams (14 oz) lighter than the birth weights of the sea-level boys. (Note that boys showed a bigger difference in birth weight than girls. Boys are more sensitive to "environmental insults"—undernutrition, toxic substances, radiation, and high altitude. No one yet knows why this is so, but the effect of altitude on birth weight is a clear example of the phenomenon.)

How does altitude affect birth weight? The air has less oxygen at high altitudes, and therefore the fetus grows more slowly in the uterus. Consequently, high-altitude newborns weigh less than sea-level babies. But do the high-altitude babies eventually catch up? To find out, I compared the height and weight at every age of the Denver girls and the Berkeley girls, and I discovered that the Denver girls did *not* catch up in weight. Denver girls weighed less at every age than Berkeley girls, even though both groups of girls were similar in height at every age. Interestingly, during the adolescent spurt, the Denver girls gained the same amount of height (8.7 in; 22.1 cm) and the same amount of weight (37 lb; 17 kg) as did the Berkeley girls. It was the growth in weight *up to* the beginning of the spurt that was slowed. This suggests that the rapid growth during the spurt is controlled independently from the growth before the spurt.

Faster Growth, Earlier Menarche

It is clear that, in general, any environmental—or genetic—factor that slows weight growth also delays menarche. Conversely, any factor that speeds up weight growth, such as ample food and fatty food, is associated with earlier menarche. For example, obese girls have menarche earlier than the average age unless their obesity is associated with pathology.

Individual girls have menarche at all different weights, though. What connects the slow or fast growth rates with the age of menarche? I had no explanation. But I did have an idea as to why body weight at the time of the first menstrual cycle could matter.

Body weight at menarche is close to adult body weight. Remember, for maintenance of the species it is a smart strategy to connect body weight and menarche. The survival of a newborn depends on the infant's birth weight, and, as noted in chapter 1, the infant's birth weight is correlated with the mother's prepregnancy weight and her weight gain during pregnancy.

What Is the Clue in Body Weight?

What did body weight represent? What was the connection between body weight and sexual maturation? When I discussed these questions with Dr. J. M. Tanner, an expert on adolescent growth at the Institute of Child Health in London, he suggested that I consult the work of Gordon C. Kennedy

of Cambridge University. I still recall the excitement of reading Kennedy's papers. He was one of the few researchers
who combined the two fields of nutrition and reproduction.
Kennedy had found that he could delay sexual maturation
(called *estrus* in nonprimate mammals) in rats indefinitely by
underfeeding them.

Kennedy stated, "Everybody knows you 'grow up' before
you mature sexually." But then he asked the important question, "How do you define being 'grown up'?" (Roger used to
say, "In the navy, they said if you are big enough, you are old
enough." Kennedy was more precise.)

Based on his research connecting body weight, food intake, and puberty in rats, Kennedy proposed that the signal
the brain receives indicating that a female is grown up
enough to reproduce successfully is related to the amount of
fat stored in the body. Kennedy also proposed that there is a
"lipostat," some sort of internal measurement of body fat
that is perceived by the hypothalamus, the part of the brain
that controls food intake and reproduction. I was so inspired
by Kennedy's work that I wrote him to ask if I might visit
him; I had the good fortune to visit him twice. I came away
from our discussions convinced that a lipostat was somehow
involved in female sexual maturation. I decided to follow this
"fatness" clue based on the idea that a critical, minimum
amount of body fat is necessary for reproduction.

After reading the human and animal body composition literature for about two years (the data for humans were very
difficult to follow because at that time there were no direct
measures of human body fat), I found that I could indeed predict a minimum weight for height necessary for menarche or
regular menstrual cycles from a fatness indicator (see chapter
6). I was cheered by this result; when you can predict, nature
is telling you something.

I am writing this about three decades after Kennedy published his lipostat idea and more than twenty-five years after
my controversial 1974 *Science* article. In 1995, I opened the
July issue of *Science* and read of Jeffrey Friedman's cloning of
the "obese" gene at Rockefeller University and of the strong

evidence for a lipostat. Friedman and other researchers reported that body fat cells produced a protein hormone called leptin (from *leptos,* the Greek word for "thin"). Leptin is perceived by special cells, called receptors, in the hypothalamus. Kennedy's paper of three decades earlier was the first publication cited in the references section of Friedman's article.

After reading Friedman's *Science* article, I sent him some of my articles on body fat, menarche, and ovulation. I also mentioned that I had visited Gordon Kennedy twice. Not long after that I was amazed to receive a call from Friedman. First he asked me about Gordon Kennedy. Then he said, "I thought you would be interested to know that you can make an infertile mouse fertile by injecting leptin," indicating that indeed leptin, and thus body fat, has a role in reproduction. (Dr. Farid Chehab of the University of California Medical Center in San Francisco published this result in *Science* in 1997: prepubertal mice—mice without fat—became pubertal after the injection of leptin. See chapter 10 for further details.)

I was present when Friedman delivered three lectures on leptin at Harvard Medical School in 1996, and he mentioned my research on the critical-fatness connection to menarche and ovulation. During the question period following one of the lectures, a man asked, "What about weight loss in men? Does it affect their reproductive ability?" "I don't know," replied Friedman. "Does anyone in the audience know?" Silence reigned in the well-filled, sizable amphitheater. I raised my hand. "I do," I said.

"As men lose weight, the first thing to go is libido—as in bulls. Then, as testosterone levels fall further, there is a loss of prostate fluid; then sperm motility and mobility are affected. Then, with an extreme, 25 percent weight loss (the men look like skeletons), sperm production is also affected. Weight gain reverses all of these effects." I was quite surprised that facts known three decades ago were new to this large medical audience, but then, this is a molecular, DNA age. I provide further details of Kennedy's research, which my collaborators and I confirmed in the rat, in chapter 6, and I discuss the increasing research on the role of leptin in reproduction in chapter 10.

A Paradox of Population Growth

A question may have occurred to you as you read about a direct link between nutrition and fertility. If undernourishment decreases fertility, how do we explain the rapid population growth of undernourished populations in developing countries? Fertility rates in many developing countries (6 to 7 children per couple) are actually far *below* the maximum human fertility (11 to 12 children per couple) found in well-nourished, noncontracepting populations. Populations of many developing countries are growing rapidly because death rates have decreased (thanks to modern public health measures) while fertility rates have remained the same. I explore this topic further in chapter 11.

Not to Neglect the Boys

My research focused on girls, but I did compare some of the adolescent events for boys who were in the same longitudinal growth studies.

Boys in the United States begin their rapid growth in height and weight simultaneously, at about age 11 on average, two years later than girls. In developing countries and historically, boys experience the spurt three years later than girls. The rapid growth continues for about three years in boys, as it does in girls, and it decelerates before *genarche*, the boys' equivalent of menarche, at about age 14.6 to 14.8. Genarche is not precisely timed because there is not a clear endpoint for boys such as the first menstrual cycle for girls. Nocturnal emissions usually begin at this time, but this event is not easy to document.

John Crawford, a pediatric endocrinologist then at Massachusetts General Hospital, suggested a possibly more precise endpoint when he urged me to study boys in detail in addition to girls. Crawford noted that apocrine sweat, which has an odor, appears at the time of genarche, so one could determine the timing of genarche by smelling the underarm sweat of boys. I declined the opportunity, and as far as I know, no one else has leaped to do it.

Why do boys start their rapid growth later, and therefore reach sexual maturation later, than girls? One possible reason may be that when girls have menarche, regular ovulatory cycles do not begin immediately. There are often irregular, anovulatory periods. Boys do not have this period of relative infertility; once they are sexually mature, sperm production is at the adult level. Later maturation for boys would therefore be an advantage for successful reproductive outcome—useful in the past, but not now! Whatever the reason, the later growth spurt for boys means that during elementary school there is a period when girls are bigger than boys at the same age. I have been amazed at the large number of men (including my husband) who remembered this time, even thirty or forty years later.

4 Eggs, Sperm, "Female Testes," and Other Fancies and Facts about the Reproductive System

I interrupt the fatness-and-fertility saga for this background chapter on some lesser-known but useful facts about human reproduction. Perhaps because human reproduction was such a taboo subject for so long (and still is to many adults), it took hundreds of years before even the elementary facts about women and men were known. This chapter relates some of this basic reproductive history, but there are still many unanswered questions.

Three hundred years ago, people had some strange ideas about the various organs of the reproductive system; for example, they believed that a human embryo was curled up in a sperm cell. I recount such ideas here because it is illuminating to know how the real facts were discovered and how long it took before those facts were accepted. I also describe some of the more wondrous mechanisms that ensure that the united egg and sperm produce a viable infant with a mixture of genes from both parents.

Discovering the Human Egg Cell

When most people think of an egg, they think of a hen's egg—about two inches long, with a smooth white or brown oval shell. For centuries, when biologists searched for the human egg, they thought it would look like a hen's egg without the shell. Naturally they didn't find it, because the human egg is far smaller. The egg is the largest cell in the female body, but it is only 0.140 millimeter (about 0.004 in) in size; about twelve human eggs would fit on the dot at the end of this sentence. If you think that is small, consider the human sperm. It is also a single cell, the smallest cell in the male body, measuring about 60 microns (0.000025 in). About 2,500 sperm in a single layer would cover the dot at the end of this sentence. Such are our beginnings.

The hen's egg is so large because it contains all the food—the yolk—needed to grow a viable chick. In contrast, the human egg contains only a small amount of fat and protein to nourish the embryo for the brief time it takes to travel down the oviduct on its way to implantation in the wall of the uterus. Once the embryo is implanted, the placenta develops and connects the growing embryo with the blood circulation of the mother for the nourishment of the fetus until birth.

As in all mammals, eggs in humans reside in the ovaries, two small, white, almond-shaped organs 3 to 5 centimeters (1.25 to 2 in) long. Each ovary weighs about 5 to 8 grams (0.2 to 0.3 oz). The ovaries hang from the broad ligament at the back of the pelvic cavity, beside the uterus. The ovaries' size is related to body size: the ovaries of a mouse are hardly bigger than a pinhead, whereas the ovary of a whale weighs about two to three pounds. But the eggs of all mammals are about the same size as the human egg.

Until the latter part of the seventeenth century, no one knew that ovaries contained eggs; as far back as the year 200, ovaries had been described as "female testes" thought to make female semen that mixed with male semen. It wasn't until about 1670 that researchers began to question the notion of female testes. Investigators then began to think that these testes were more like the ovaries of birds; they could see that the hen's ovaries had developing eggs in them because the eggs were so large. In 1672 the Dutch physician Regnier de Graaf proved that the human female "testis" was really an ovary; he discovered ovarian follicles, now known as Graafian follicles. De Graaf thought the whole developing follicle, which is large and can be seen as a bulge on the surface of the ovary, was the human egg, but it isn't. It took another century and a half to see the tiny human egg cell contained within the follicle.

In 1677 Dutch scientist Antonie von Leeuwenhoek discovered sperm cells. He concluded that a rudimentary embryo lay inside the sperm and that the female uterus—which everybody did find while they were looking for the egg—was just a place of nourishment for the sperm while it developed. Leeuwenhoek denied the existence of eggs in mammals altogether.

Many investigators kept looking for the elusive egg until 1827, when Karl von Baer, an Estonian embryologist, noticed a minute, yellowish spot floating freely in a Graafian follicle. Curious, he opened the follicle with the point of a knife and was astonished to observe what looked like a tiny mammalian egg floating in the fluid. Placing it under a microscope, he realized from his careful, earlier observations of developing embryos in the oviduct that it was the mammalian egg. He wrote, "It is truly wonderful and surprising to be able to demonstrate to the eye, by so simple a procedure, a thing which has been sought so persistently and discussed ad nauseam in every textbook of physiology as insoluble."

As often happens in science, little attention was paid to Baer's papers on his discovery. At a meeting in 1828, no one even spoke to him of his finding. But one foreign visitor asked Baer if it would be possible to have a demonstration of the mammalian ovum. It was arranged on the spot by sacrificing a local dog. A group of young biologists also attended this demonstration of an egg inside a follicle of the dog, and the truth about the mammalian egg was carried to the labs all over Europe. It had taken nearly two thousand years to find it.

PRODUCTION OF GAMETES: EGGS AND SPERM

Egg and sperm cells are called *gametes* (from the Greek words for wife and husband). Nature is lavish in the production of gametes. At about the fifth month of development in the uterus, a female fetus has about seven million *oogonia* (cells that will become egg cells, or *oocytes*). Production of oocytes in the female fetus ends by the seventh month of gestation, never to be resumed. At birth a baby girl has about a million oocytes in her ovaries. By menarche, at about age 12.5, she has about 500,000 oocytes; about half of the original oocytes have degenerated. Only about 400 of these oocytes are ever ovulated.[1]

Why the human female has so many egg cells is not known. Perhaps it is so because we are descended from fish. Female fish have to release millions of eggs into the water, where the eggs are fertilized by the male. The developing embryos are exposed to numerous predators and hazards so that only a small number of the millions of the eggs released and fertilized survive to adulthood.

Each cell in the body of the human female has 46 chromosomes—22 pairs of somatic (body) chromosomes and two sex chromosomes, X and X. Males also have 46 chromosomes in their body cells. They, too, have 22 pairs of somatic chromosomes, but they have one X and one Y sex chromosome. The genetic pair XX of the sex chromosomes codes for the creation of ovaries in the developing embryo; it's a girl. The genetic pair XY codes for development of testes in the developing embryo; it's a boy. The presence of the Y chromosome is necessary for maleness. When Y is lacking, the embryo XO develops as a female, though not a normal female.

Before an egg or sperm is ready for fertilization in a sexually mature woman or man, the number of chromosomes has to be reduced by half. The reason is simple: the egg and sperm will unite their chromosome number after fertilization, and the total number has to be 46, 22 pairs plus two sex chromosomes. The female contributes 23 chromosomes plus an X, and the male contributes 23 chromosomes plus an X or a Y to

1. This number is estimated from a human reproductive span of about forty years, from the age of 12.5 to menopause at age 52, the average span for a well-nourished woman, assuming the ovulation of one egg per month and no pregnancies.

the newly fertilized egg. Thus both parents contribute their genes to the start of a new human being.

Reducing the chromosome number in the egg and sperm by half before they are ready for fertilization involves a rather complicated process called *meiosis* or *reduction division*. During the first stage of meiosis, the chromosomes come together in pairs, one chromosome originally from the mother and one originally from the father. The precise lineup of the genes on the chromosomes allows the genes to cross over from one to another, so that the 23 new pairs of chromosomes become a new mixture of maternal and paternal genes.

The matched pairs of chromosomes then duplicate themselves. At this stage the cell that will become the egg is called the primary oocyte, and the cell that will become the sperm is called the primary spermatocyte. After the duplication, the second stage of meiosis takes place. Two cell divisions occur, yielding the gametes; each of the gametes has only 23 chromosomes, one from each of the original pairs. The timing of this second stage is quite different for the egg than for the sperm.

Each of the 23 maternal chromosomes and each of the 23 paternal chromosomes is sorted independently into the egg and sperm, and fertilization of the egg by the sperm restores the number so that there are 46 chromosomes in the developing embryo. The number of possible combinations of chromosomes is 2 to the 23rd power, or 8,388,608 possible combinations. That is why resemblances between parents and children (or lack of them) are so varied and sometimes so surprising.

Two-Stage Ovulation of an Egg

By the time a baby girl is born, all the oogonia (early egg cells with 46 chromosomes) have completed the first division, reducing the number of chromosomal pairs in half. The resulting cells, which reside in the infant's ovaries, have 23 chromosomes each and are called secondary oocytes. But, as if frozen in time, these oocytes remain suspended in that mid-meiosis stage until a girl reaches sexual maturity, at age 12.6 on average. At that time, only one egg completes the second division and is ovulated. Each egg to be ovulated in each month thereafter does not complete reduction division until *right before it is ovulated*. Thus some eggs do not complete reduction division until thirty or forty years after starting the process before birth. That explains why women over 40 are more likely to have babies with Down's syndrome, which is caused by an extra number 23 chromosome. Chromosomal abnormalities in general arise more frequently in the eggs that complete the reduction division late in the reproductive life span. I could find no explanation for this time-staggered preparation of an egg for ovulation. Apparently no one has remarked on it, though it is so different from the sperm.

Usually only one egg ovulates at a time. How or why a particular egg is selected for ovulation is still not known. Normally a group of oocytes starts developing, but only one continues while the others degenerate. When two eggs ovulate, as sometimes happens, fraternal twins develop. When one fertilized egg splits into two, identical twins develop. The tendency to have twins is inherited.

Uninterrupted Production of Sperm

Sperm cells do not have the interrupted development in reduction division and maturation found in the egg. Primitive sperm cells, or *primary spermatocytes,* start their further development at genarche, which occurs at about age 14.5 for boys in the United States. They then complete the first stage of reduction division by reducing their chromosome number in half, to 23. Each of these sperm cells then divides again into four sperm, each with 23 chromosomes.

As one physiologist has described it, on reaching puberty the human male continues to make sperm monotonously for the duration of his life, so sperm cells are normally always available. The human ejaculate has a volume of 2 to 5 ml (about 0.1 to 0.2 fl oz) and contains from 60 to 100 million sperm per milliliter.

Mammalian testes, including human testes, are sensitive to temperature. Oddly, sperm production cannot take place if the testis is exposed to the normal temperature, 98.6°F, of the interior of the body. How or why this temperature intolerance evolved is unknown. Since they can't be inside the body, the testes hang outside the body in the scrotal sac, where the temperature is slightly lower than inside the body. The testes normally descend into the scrotal sac before birth. The scrotal sac is constructed to stay cool; it has no subcutaneous fat, and it has numerous sweat glands to dissipate heat. High fevers in men can be followed by a temporary loss of mature sperm. Apparently, soaking in excessively hot baths can have the same effect.

CYCLICITY DEFINES THE FEMALE

In contrast to the male's steady production of sperm, cyclicity defines the female reproductive system. Most females, whether birds or mammals (including women), have a cyclical pattern of ovulation. The domestic hen has the shortest ovarian cycle: she lays an egg once a day. Fortunately the human cycle is longer; women in the reproductive years ovulate in a 28-day cycle, with some variation, plus or minus two or three days. There is no evidence that this cycle is related to the phases of the moon, though it has been fancied.

In most nonprimate mammals the cyclic period of ovulation is timed with a period of sexual receptivity called an estrous period (known popularly as being "in heat"). Rats and mice have a very short cycle, ovulating multiple eggs every four or five days, except when the cycles are interrupted by a pregnancy, which also is short—just three weeks; hence the large numbers of rats and mice. Cows, mares, and pigs have estrous periods at 21-day intervals. Pigs ovulate about a dozen eggs every 21 days, hence the large number of pigs. Dogs and cats have only two or three estrous periods each year.

For many wild animals, the estrous period is so timed that food will be plentiful when the young are weaned. Lower primates—apes and monkeys—have cyclic fluctuations in sexual activity in the wild, but not in captivity. The human female can mate on any day of the ovarian cycle, but the egg can be fertilized only if ovulation has occurred and the egg is still in the ampulla (an enlarged area) of the fallopian tube. No outward sign of ovulation occurs in women as it does in some mammals, including lower primates. However, some women experience a slight pain, which they recognize as ovulation, in the middle of the monthly cycle. Most women show a slight but distinct rise in their basal body temperature just after ovulation. This increase in temperature does not occur consistently in all women, and it can be brought on by infections and other external factors, so it is not always a reliable indicator of ovulation.

Hypothalamic Control of Cyclic Ovulation

All the physiological and behavioral controls that are coordinated with the preparation of the egg and eventual cyclic ovulation in women are regulated by the central nervous system. As figure 5 below shows, the hypothalamus, which is part of the third ventricle of the brain, controls and orchestrates the mechanisms involved.

It is the hypothalamus that sends signals to the next regulator, the *pituitary gland,* which is an endocrine organ. Endocrine glands pour their secretions directly into the bloodstream, where they are picked up by receptors in the target organs. The pituitary gland regulates the function of the ovaries or the testes, the adrenal gland, the thyroid gland, and the other endocrine organs of the body. The ovaries and the testes also secrete hormones; the follicles of the ovaries produce estrogen and progesterone, the most important female hormones. Cells in the testes produce testosterone, the most important male hormone. All these hormones are steroids, derived from cholesterol.

You should be surprised that the hypothalamus is the master regulator of the endocrine system; everybody else was. For decades, everybody thought the pituitary gland was the master gland, the one that ran the works. What's more, the notion that cells of the central nervous system could release hormones into the bloodstream was unthinkable. Nerve cells were known to transfer information by transmitting substances at a synapse, the point of contact of a nerve cell process to other nerve cells, or a body part, such as muscle. But it was an unorthodox idea that nerve cells in the hypothalamus could synthesize hormones. Yet that's what British researcher Geoffrey Harris discovered about five decades ago. The hypothalamus synthesizes hormones and releases them into the capillary blood vessels, from which they flow into a special blood system, the portal blood vessels, to the pituitary gland.

When researchers were still skeptical that nerve cells could make hormones, Harris showed, in a clinching experiment, that if he inserted a plate across the cut stalk of the portal vessels of the hypothalamus and the pituitary gland of a female animal, the animal did not ovulate. Blood vessels from the hypothalamus had to be connected to the pituitary gland for ovulation to occur because this unique portal circulation carried the signals to the pituitary to release the two principal hormones necessary for ovulation, follicle-stimulating hormone (FSH) and luteinizing hormone (LH).

The hypothalamus weighs only about 10 grams (about 0.4 oz); the whole human brain weighs about 1,200 to 1,400 grams (42 to 50 oz). Those 10 grams control not only reproduction but also food and water intake, sleep, body temperature, and emotions. The hypothalamus receives messages from the higher centers of the brain. Reproduction and the other functions are thus clued into the environment by messages from the higher centers on such external factors as light and temperature.

A RELEASING HORMONE SAYS "GO"

"Releasing hormones," which stimulate the secretion of hormones in the pituitary gland, are secreted into the bloodstream by the hypothalamus. Gonadotropin-releasing hor-

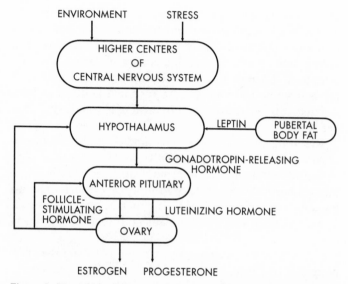

Figure 5. Hypothalamic control of reproduction. The hypothalamus, part of the third ventricle of the brain, controls the hormonal secretions that lead to ovulation and to regularly timed menstrual cycles. Pulses of gonadotropin-releasing hormone (GnRH) secreted by the hypothalamus cause the pituitary gland to release follicle-stimulating hormone (FSH), which controls the growth of an ovarian follicle (specialized cells that encase an egg), and luteinizing hormone (LH), which controls ovulation (the midcycle release of the egg). In the first half of the cycle the growing follicle secretes estrogen. This hormone modulates the activity of the pituitary gland and stimulates the growth of the breasts and of the lining of the uterus. After ovulation, the ruptured follicle becomes the corpus luteum, which secretes progesterone, a hormone that promotes the vascularization (increase of blood vessels) of the uterine lining in preparation for the implanting of a fertilized egg. If the egg is not fertilized, estrogen and progesterone levels fall, and the uterine lining is shed—menstruation occurs. Hypothalamic function can be affected by signals from the higher centers of the brain, such as stress. We now know that the hypothalamus also receives signals on the amount of body fat from the recently discovered hormone, leptin, which is secreted by body fat. Loss of a critical amount of body fat disrupts the normal, pulsatile release of GnRH by the hypothalamus.

mone (GnRH) is the controlling hormone for reproduction; it activates the pituitary gland to produce the cascade of hormones that result in ovulation. GnRH is secreted in pulses. When the pulses reach a certain frequency and concentration, the rest of the reproductive system signals "go" for ovulation. The human gene encoding GnRH has been isolated: it is located on the short arm of chromosome number 8.

Releasing hormones consist of simple peptides (chains of amino acids) in various sizes; GnRH is a small peptide consisting of ten amino acids. Amino acids are the building blocks of proteins. All proteins in all species, from bacteria to humans, are constructed from combinations of the same set of twenty amino acids. The fundamental alphabet of proteins is at least 2 billion years old.

Sexually mature girls and women normally have the "go" pattern of GnRH pulses that results in monthly ovulation. As researchers discovered in the mid-1970s, prepubertal girls have a low-level, "non-go" pattern of GnRH pulses, differing in frequency and concentration of hormone from the mature pattern. As girls experience the adolescent growth spurt, the prepubertal pattern changes to the "go" pattern.

What signals the hypothalamus to shift gears to "go"? One important clue for me is the fact that mature women who have amenorrhea (absence of cycles) because of moderate weight loss also have prepubertal, "non-go" pulse patterns of GnRH; these patterns return to "go" once weight is gained. The women's weight loss and gain were in a range that indicated loss or gain of body fat.

Illustrating the control by the hypothalamus even more clearly, Swedish scientist Sven Nillius was able, in 1977, to reverse the non-go GnRH pattern in adult women who had anorexia and amenorrhea. He did this by continuously injecting pulsed GnRH into the bloodstream; in time the pituitary gland responded by secreting normal levels of FSH and LH. Thus, the pituitary-ovary axis had been ready to go all along, but the hypothalamus had said no.

By now you know that a big question was still unanswered: What signals the hypothalamus that it's time to establish the "go" pattern of GnRH pulses? We know the pituitary gland waits on the hypothalamus, but what is communicated to the hypothalamus, and by what means? Until the discovery of leptin, there were no definite answers to that question. Some researchers simply said that the hypothalamus "matures," and feedbacks to the hypothalamus from the ovary change. Feedbacks from the ovaries do change, but scientists had yet to explain what it meant for the hypothalamus to "mature."

I hypothesized that something informs the hypothalamus that the body is now grown up enough to maintain a successful pregnancy, signaling that it is OK to begin the warm-up for ovulatory cycles. Recall the example I gave above; if girls or women lose weight so that their body composition reverts to the prepubertal ratio of high lean mass to low body fat, the GnRH secretion also reverts to the prepubertal, "non-go" pulse pattern. Weight gain restores pulsatile secretion of GnRH to adult levels and frequency.

If we accept the hypothesis about the hypothalamus, the question then becomes, what can be the signals? One possibility is that body fat—or adipose tissue, to use the medical term—secretes substances into the bloodstream that inform the hypothalamus that the body has achieved a "grown up" composition. It is now known that leptin, a hormone made by body fat, is indeed one of those substances. Leptin controls food intake and energy metabolism, and, to my great pleasure, it has been found to play a major role in reproductive ability. For details see chapter 10, which is devoted entirely to leptin.

Another possible signal to the hypothalamus is metabolic rate, the rate of heat production in the body. As the ratio of lean mass to body fat changes, metabolic rate also changes. An associated signal could be changes in body temperature; leaner women often have abnormal temperature control.

Whatever the signals, by about age 12.5, on average, the pulsatile release of GnRH leads to the cyclical release of FSH and LH by the pituitary gland, resulting in the monthly menstrual cycle (note that *menses* comes from the Greek word for month). There are two functional phases of the menstrual cycle: the first is the follicular phase, when one of a group of follicles begins to enlarge and mature; the second is the luteal phase, after ovulation, when the egg is released from the follicle and enters the fallopian tube on its way to the uterus.

At the start of each monthly cycle (the first day of the menstrual period is day one), an increase in the release of FSH by the pituitary gland stimulates a crop of growing follicles to undergo further growth. Then most of the follicles degenerate while one continues to grow; how the lucky follicle is chosen is not known. Cells within the chosen follicle begin to secrete estrogen. The rising estrogen levels in the bloodstream cause the glands in the lining of the uterus, the endometrium, to begin growing in preparation of receiving the fertilized egg. The rising level of estrogen eventually triggers a sharp rise in the level of LH released by the pituitary gland; this results in ovulation, the release of the egg from the follicle. Ovulation is not explosive; the egg, which by then floats freely in the fluid of the follicle, passes out passively. Ovulation usually occurs about fourteen to fifteen days after the start of the menstrual cycle, but it can occur anywhere from the ninth to the seventeenth day due to variability in the length of the follicular, preovulatory phase.

Transport of the Egg

After all these fancy arrangements to get the egg out of the follicle, you would think that the oviduct—the passage it must travel to the uterus—would be safely attached to the ovary. In many animals, including rodents, dogs, and cats, it is. But in humans the oviduct—the fallopian tube—is separate from the ovary. Once the egg leaves the follicle, it is directed toward the fallopian tube by the maneuvering of the funnel-shaped free end of the oviduct, which has fingerlike projections, called the fimbria, that are covered with cilia (small, hairlike projections). As a result of the movements of the fimbria over the ovary's surface at the time of ovulation and the currents caused by the beating of the cilia, the egg is captured and carried by the currents into the depths of the oviduct. This is rather a casual way of getting the egg under way. Some eggs actually miss the oviduct and fall into the body cavity, but fortunately this is a rare occurrence (fig. 6).

Once in the oviduct, the egg is transported by the beating of the cilia and by the muscular contractions of the oviduct walls, both controlled by estrogen and progesterone. In most mammals the period of sexual receptivity, estrus, begins several hours before ovulation, so when the egg gets to the ampulla, the site of fertilization, the spermatazoa are waiting for it.

FERTILIZATION OF THE EGG

In women, unlike in other animals, there is no relation between coitus and ovulation, so the egg usually has to await the arrival of the sperm. Spermatazoa reach the ampulla of the fallopian tube five minutes after they are deposited in the vagina. The egg cannot wait long; its fertile life is brief, probably under twenty-four hours. Spermatazoa also are believed to have a short fertile life, not more than twenty-four hours. According to some researchers, however, sperm may remain motile in the reproductive tract for up to a week but probably retain the capacity to fertilize the egg in the fallopian tube for only three or four days.

Tens of millions, or even hundreds of millions, of spermatazoa are deposited in the vagina, but those that reach the egg number only a hundred to a few thousand. Only one spermatazoa works its way through the gelatinous coats that enclose the egg. When it does, all other sperm are excluded. The fertilized egg then makes its way down the fallopian tube to the uterus.

The egg–sperm transport system can break down at several points. The most common mishap is an ectopic pregnancy in the fallopian tube, which occurs when the egg is fertilized but is not moved on to the uterus. Instead, it becomes attached to the wall of the oviduct, and a tubal preg-

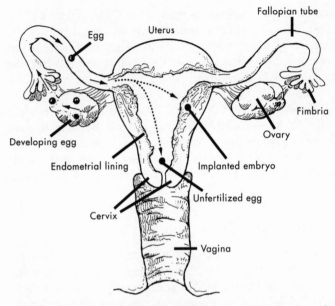

Figure 6. The female reproductive system (front view). Note how the egg is casually dropped from the ovary to the unattached fimbria of the fallopian tube. Copyright © by Harriet Greenfield. From R. L. Barbieri, A. D. Domar, and K. R. Loughlin, *Six Steps to Increased Fertility* (New York: Simon and Schuster, 2000), 48.

nancy results. Such a pregnancy cannot continue and requires surgical removal. Inflammatory disease of the ovarian tubes is the most frequent cause of tubal pregnancy.

Considering the complexity of the changes culminating in the ovulation of the egg, it would seem reasonable that once the egg was out of the follicle, the follicle would just collapse, and that would be the end of it. The follicle does collapse, but then it changes into an endocrine gland called the *corpus luteum,* literally the yellow body, whose color is caused by the accumulation of lipids, or fatty substances. Proliferating within the corpus luteum are lutein cells that secrete progesterone, a steroid hormone that plays an important role in

EGGS, SPERM, "FEMALE TESTES"   53

maintaining pregnancy once the egg has been fertilized. Progesterone regulates the lining of the uterus, or *endometrium,* so that a fertilized egg can be implanted and develop, and it inhibits muscular contractions of the uterus that might threaten the egg's ability to remain attached to the uterine wall. If the egg has been fertilized, it is implanted in the enriched lining of the uterus on about the twenty-second or twenty-third day of the menstrual cycle. If the egg is not fertilized, it disintegrates and passes from the body; then the corpus luteum begins to regress, the capillaries of the endometrium collapse, and the cells begin to atrophy.

Shedding the Endometrium: Menstruation

Menstruation, the shedding of the endometrium, then occurs as a result of a drop in the levels of progesterone and, in particular, estrogen. Each menstrual cycle culminates in menstrual bleeding, and the first day of menstruation is considered day one of the cycle. Like everything else in this amazing process, the shedding of the endometrium is a complicated affair. It contains unique spiral blood vessels that appear coiled; when the endometrium contracts, it causes the spiral blood vessels to kink, decreasing their blood supply. Because they lack blood supply, the capillaries break down, spurting tiny drops of blood into the tissue of the endometrium. Ultimately these small hemorrhages coalesce, and the blood is discharged into the uterine cavity. Although the blood clots as it exudes from the blood vessels, the menstrual flow is usually liquefied as a result of *lysis* (breakdown) of the clots while they are in the vagina. Sometimes large clots remain because the bleeding is occurring too rapidly for the clot to lyse in the vagina, but this is of no consequence for health.

Normally only a small amount of blood is lost during menstruation, less than 50 milliliters (2 fl oz). Bleeding usually lasts about four to five days; it is profuse the first three days and then tapers off. Once the shedding of the lining, which extends to the basal cells of the endometrium, is complete, the bleeding ceases, and the endometrium starts to grow again, including new spiral arteries, preparing for the next cycle.

Although menstruation usually occurs about every four weeks, the regularity of the rhythm varies widely. Studies of the cycle among large groups of women of all ages from menarche to menopause show that a regular 28-day cycle, with variability of plus or minus two or three days, is characteristic only during the peak years of reproductive ability, from about ages 20 to 35. Cycles can be very irregular after menarche, the first cycle, and they become increasingly irregular again in the years before the menopause, in the mid- and late 40s. (Menopause is now at about age 52 on average, in American women.) Menstrual cycles also can be anovulatory, without ovulation at all. The shedding of the lining in that case is the result of the drop in estrogen. Many of the cycles soon after menarche are anovulatory, as are cycles shortly before menopause.

Menstruation occurs only in primates. The vaginal bleeding that occurs in other mammalian species, such as the dog, is physiologically different and associated with the engorgement of the genital organs that takes place at estrus, which occurs at the time of ovulation. The bleeding is just the opposite of menstruation, which takes place two weeks after ovulation if fertilization of the egg has not taken place.

WHY MENSTRUATION?

Why do primates have menstruation, shedding the lining of the uterus, instead of quietly absorbing the enlarged glandular cells of the uterus, as many lower animals do? One possible explanation may be the fact that the endometrial cells shed by primates can survive if they become implanted elsewhere in the body. Endometriosis, the troublesome condition that renders many women temporarily or even permanently sterile, develops when pieces of the endometrium enter the body cavity and attach to the outside of the ovary or other abdominal organs. These endometrial cells then respond to the changes in ovarian hormones as if they were still in the lining of the uterus.

In fact, the spiral arteries that are unique to the endometrium were first seen in a piece of the endometrium that was transplanted to the eye of a monkey. The small grafts were placed just behind the clear cornea, and they received their blood supply from vessels that grew into them from the iris of the eye. When menstruation occurred in the uterus, it occurred at the same time in the eye grafts, ran the same course, and ceased at the same time. J. E. Markee, the researcher who did the grafts at Stanford University, could observe through a microscope the blanching of the tissues due to the shutting off of the blood flow by contraction of the coiled arteries. The coiled arteries have never been found in nonmenstruating animals.

Although the anatomical details of the menstrual cycle are awesomely complex, the nerve cells of the hypothalamus have the ultimate control, so the menstrual cycle can be changed or turned off by environmental factors including emotional stress and even changes in time zones. For example, flight attendants who travel long distances east to west and thus cross different time zones report changes in their menstrual cycle. Presumably exposure to light is involved, but the mechanism is not yet known. And as we now know, the physical stress of being underweight or too lean can affect the length of the cycle or turn it off completely. Everything should be in peak condition for the uterus to receive a fertilized egg and start its development. The control system indicates, if you can't do it right, don't do it at all.

PHEROMONES

Women who live communally—in a dormitory, for example —eventually have their menstrual cycles at the same time. This odd phenomenon was first explained by the action of a special type of hormone called *pheromones*. Pheromones are unique because they are released into the air and then absorbed from the air. But they are odorless. You cannot smell a pheromone; you just unconsciously react to it. These odorless compounds can change the physiology and behavior of the women exposed to them. Humans and animals both release pheromones, but fortunately they are species specific.

When I first learned of synchronized menstrual cycles, the idea of pheromones was still controversial. Did they exist or didn't they? I thought it very possible that they did because, in the prehistoric past, there would have been a good reason for women's menstrual cycles to be synchronized. There may have been selection in the prehistoric past for women who were sensitive to pheromones, because women who have their menstrual cycles at the same time might also tend to ovulate at the same time and thus to have their pregnancies at the same time. Then, if a mother died, her infant could be nursed by a mother whose infant had died. In those times of high infant and maternal mortality, this could have been an important mechanism for the survival of the species.

In more recent times, these pheromones could wreak havoc in a harem. The sheik obviously could not solve the problem by adding a new wife because, after an interval, she would cycle with the other wives. The only solution would be to build a new palace for each new wife, an expensive proposition. Perhaps that's one of the reasons monogamy became popular.

That women indeed produce odorless compounds from their armpits that affect the menstrual cycles of other women was recently confirmed by Kathleen Stern and Martha McClintock of the University of Chicago. Their methodology was admirably direct. Donor women wore cotton pads in their axillae (armpits) for at least eight hours. Each pad was then cut into four sections to be used for exposure to the recipient women. Recipients were first studied for one baseline menstrual cycle without exposure to the pads. The donors were checked to be in hormonally distinct phases of the menstrual cycle, either in the late follicular phase (before ovulation) or at ovulation.

Pads from the donors were wiped daily under the noses of women recipients during two complete menstrual cycles.

Half the women received "wipes" with follicular compounds daily, and half received "wipes" with ovulatory compounds daily. Then, the compounds administered were reversed for each woman. None of the women was aware that the experiment was on pheromones. "Don't wash your face for the next six hours" was their only instruction.

Results were clear-cut: odorless compounds from the armpits of women in the late follicular phase of the cycle accelerated the preovulatory surge of LH necessary for ovulation and shortened the menstrual cycles of the recipient women. In contrast, axillary compounds from the same donors collected later in the cycle, at ovulation, had the opposite effect: the pheromones delayed the LH surge of the recipients and lengthened their menstrual cycles.

Only the follicular phase of the cycle (before ovulation) was regulated—shortened by the follicular compounds and lengthened by the ovulatory compounds—suggesting, the authors wrote, that there are separate pheromones that have opposite effects on a woman's ovulation. One pheromone speeded up the follicles' rate of maturation, shortening the cycle; the other altered the hormonal threshold necessary for the LH surge that precedes ovulation, lengthening the cycle.

Most medical textbooks state that the normal luteal phase (after ovulation) has a fixed length of fourteen days. But Stern and McClintock found that the luteal phase could vary in length as well. My colleagues and I found such variations in length when we studied the effects of physical activity on the menstrual cycles among athletes.

Although ovarian-dependent pheromones are now confirmed to be out there in the air, Stern and McClintock caution that because the donors and recipients in their study were healthy young women, ages 20 to 35, at the peak of the reproductive years, the results cannot be generalized to women in other age groups. Further research will explore whether older or younger women also emit pheromones and whether other reproductive events, such as puberty or menopause or intervals between births, are also affected. Because I am always curious about a possible role for female body fat, I wonder whether a fatter woman produces more pheromones than a leaner one, and whether a fatter recipient is more sensitive to pheromones than a leaner one.

And what would happen if a man wore a pad under his armpit for eight hours and then wiped it under the nose of his girlfriend daily during her menstrual cycle? Or vice versa for the man daily at any time? I doubt funding will be available to find out.

5 Historical Guesses

What Hastened or Slowed Menarche?

Over the centuries no one predicted when a girl would have her first menstrual cycle, but it was not for lack of interest. When I looked up references to menarche in a medical library, I found countless records dating back to Aristotle in the third century B.C. There seemed to be an obsession about menarche. Doctors, philosophers, explorers, and educators wrote or reported about the age of menarche in various populations, and some of the writers had weird ideas of what hastened or slowed the age reported, as I will recount. This interest is especially surprising considering the age-old taboo against mentioning the menstrual cycle and other details of female reproduction.

One possible reason for the strong interest in the age of menarche is that in many developing countries girls are considered marriageable as soon as they have had menarche. Consequently, such girls have to be sequestered lest some male "get at them." In some South Asian communities, for example, girls must leave school once they have had their first menstrual cycle, even if they are just a few months short of their graduation or certificate. Their parents probably don't know that as the hoped-for rise in economic standards in these communities is attained, menarche will occur earlier because girls will be better nourished and will grow more quickly. If the custom of removing girls from school is maintained, girls will be less educated than their predecessors—a rather ironic result of better times.

Another possible reason for the strong interest in age of menarche in the past is the lack of a similarly defining event for boys. There is no way to tell for sure what is going on in boys at the same age, other than noting that their voice is breaking. When a boy's voice changes from soprano to tenor or bass, it is understandably much less of a sexual event than the first menstrual cycle. Besides, boys are not married off when their voices change; in the past they might have been dismissed from the choir, or, in some unfortunate cases centuries ago, castrated in advance to maintain the soprano voice.

LIKE GIRLS, BOYS SHOW LONG-TERM TREND TOWARD EARLIER SEXUAL DEVELOPMENT

Because the time of boys' first nocturnal emission is not easy to document, especially historically, the records of voice change for boys are especially valuable. These records show that changes in the age at which the boys' voice breaks are consistent with the long-term trend to an earlier menarche observed for girls. In mid-eighteenth-century Leipzig, for example, the average age of voice change was 18, according to records kept during the years 1727–1749 by the chorus of Johann Sebastian Bach. Currently the average age for well-nourished boys is 13.5 (one year before genarche). Historians noted that when economic times worsened, the age of voice change became later, just as the age of menarche became later for girls. When economic times improved, the ages of menarche and voice change became earlier again. No one apparently asked why there was such a close correlation. Occasionally there were vague references to the level of nutrition being better or worse, but there was no explanation of why that would matter.

Does Sweet Music Hasten Menarche?

They did, however, have some dazzling ideas in the past of what could affect the age of menarche. Sweet music, for instance, was supposed to hasten the age of menarche. This notion was actually tested experimentally in 1844, as reported by the chief of the obstetrics hospital in Paris, Dr. M. A. Raciborski. Members of the Paris Philharmonic Orchestra went to the Paris zoo (Jardin des Plantes) and assembled behind a curtain near the elephant cage. The orchestra performed the Dance in B Minor from Gluck's *Iphegénie en Tauride.* The elephants' reactions to the music were carefully noted— the male preferred the clarinet solos, the female the bassoon solos. After this single exposure to music, it was found that these elephants matured at age 16 and 17, eight years younger than elephants in the wild.

It's not very probable that the elephants' earlier maturation was caused by exposure to Gluck's music, lovely as it is. It is much more likely that the elephants matured earlier because elephants in captivity have more food, and more regular food, than elephants in the wild; moreover, as Charles Darwin observed, animals in captivity do not have to expend energy to get the food. In fact, many animals in captivity mature earlier and are more fertile than their relatives in the wild.

Dr. Raciborski reported the music experiment without endorsement. He thought undernutrition was one of the most important factors delaying the age of menarche among his female hospital patients. Menarche among those women often occurred as late as age 28.

Doctors who collected menarcheal ages of foreign populations for comparison with local data also noted the importance of nutrition. Black slave girls in the West Indies, where food was poor and physical work hard, reportedly had menarche at about age 16, similar in age to white English working-class girls, who were also relatively undernourished. Currently, black girls living in poor areas of Africa also have a late age of menarche, 15 to 16 years, whereas well-

nourished white girls in the same areas have menarche between ages 12.5 and 13. Thus, there is little evidence for the
idea that black girls have menarche genetically earlier than
white girls.

Also, girls in hot climates do not necessarily have an early
age of menarche. Again, nutritional level seems to override
any effects of climate. Poorly nourished girls in hot, rural areas of India have menarche at about age 15 to 16, whereas
well-nourished girls in Indian cities have menarche at about
age 12.5, like girls in the United States.

Exposure to Sexuality

In Victorian times, an unusual influence thought to affect the
age of menarche was exposure to sexuality, or what we might
now call sexual harassment—in particular, the "unwelcome
advances" of upper-class men to their household servants. A
nineteenth-century doctor considered the proposition and
decided there was nothing in it. His reasoning is illuminating:
If exposure to sexuality caused early puberty, we should find
puberty occurring earlier in the laboring and destitute females of large towns than among the upper classes. But, he
continued, we find that the reverse is true: women in the upper classes have menarche earlier than those in the lower
classes, sometimes by as much as sixteen to eighteen months.
Yet surely virtue is not less cherished in the upper classes?
Continuing his argument, the doctor pointed out that young
females employed in shops, factories, and houses as domes-
tics are "constantly in 'unavoidable collision' with the opposite sex a grade above them," and many of the latter employ
artifices to bring ruin and disgrace upon the creatures they
should protect. "It is a wonder that any escape childhood
uncontaminated," he remarked. Yet these poor, sexually ha-
rassed girls had menarche later than the virtuous upper
classes.

A current variant of this notion is that the jazzy atmo-
sphere of cities, with all their bright lights and other stimuli
(usually unspecified), results in an earlier age of menarche.

No evidence supports this idea, either. Girls in cities eat more and better food than girls in rural areas do, so they grow faster than the rural girls. (I was surprised to learn that girls in rural areas were less well nourished than city girls, because I thought they could eat more eggs and milk and grains. But the farmers must sell their produce, so their daughters are less well fed than city girls.)

Also in the nineteenth century, Belgian statistician and Royal astronomer Adolphe Quetelet quoted ages of menarche for Danish girls as 15.7 years for blondes and 17.54 years for brunettes, one of the more esoteric pieces of information on menarche in the literature. Quetelet had a deep understanding of the importance of physical growth in relation to menarche, so he would not have listed hair color as a cause of a delayed or early menarche. The unexplained correlation was just one more bit of information people collected, hoping it would fit in somehow to enable prediction.

GENETIC INFLUENCE

One influence on menarche that *is* now well established is genetic. Identical twins differ in their age of menarche by only two or three months; in contrast, sisters and nonidentical twins differ by about a year. Mothers and daughters have more closely related ages of menarche than do unrelated women, who differ in age of menarche by about eighteen months.

One reason for the influence of genetics on menarche is simple: children inherit their growth rate. Some children are genetic fast growers, and some are genetic slow growers, though they have the same parents and the same environmental influences. We still do not know what determines this normal genetic difference. Fast growers eat more; but what makes them eat more than slow growers?

Animal experiments have shown that it is not possible to convert a genetic slow grower into a fast grower; "food intake," the amount of food a person normally eats, is apparently also genetically determined. Of course, it is possible to convert a genetic fast grower into a slow grower by making an environmental change, that is, by decreasing the amount of food available.

Of all the ideas of what influenced the age of menarche, only one made sense to me. This was the "lipostat" theory of Gordon C. Kennedy of Cambridge University, which I discuss in chapter 3. Inspired by Kennedy, my question became, What was the body composition of a girl at menarche— how much body fat did she have? That was one question about menarche that apparently had not been answered—or asked—in the past.

6   Predicting Menarche

Critical Fatness

A girl's adolescent growth spurt always precedes menarche, and it is a true spurt—a speed-up of growth rates. All of a sudden, at age 9 to 9.5, a girl begins to gain height and then weight. (See the sharp rise in weight gain shown in chapter 3, figure 3.) These rapid rates of growth in the three-year interval to menarche transform a child into almost a grown-up. The spurt in weight is particularly large; a girl starts at about 66 pounds, on average, and three years later, at menarche, weighs 103 pounds, on average. She is a child of four feet six inches tall, on average, at the start and reaches five feet two inches tall at menarche, on average. Accompanying these rapid growth changes are the hormonal and reproductive-system changes that culminate in the first menstrual cycle.

Growth rates in height and weight begin to slow down about six months before menarche, but girls continue to grow in height and weight until they are 16 to 18 years old. When girls in our study finished growing at age 16 to 18, they averaged 65 inches (165 cm) in height and had gained another 22 pounds (10 kg), weighing 125 pounds (57 kg), on average.

Note that a girl's final height is not related to her height at menarche. Early maturers are shorter at menarche than are late maturers, but they all have the same average height when they finish growing; the height attained at maturity is unrelated to the speed with which it is reached. But the late maturers—girls who start the adolescent spurt at about age 11 or 12 instead of 9 or 10 and who grow at slower rates during the spurt—are leaner than the plumper early maturers when their growth is completed.

Growth of the Reproductive Organs

More than just height and weight change in these years of adolescent growth and transformation. The breasts and all the reproductive organs—the ovaries, the uterus, the fallopian tubes (which carry the egg from the ovary to the uterus), and the vagina—increase markedly in size, and the female pelvis becomes wider. These changes are only partly completed at the time of menarche; the mature adult size of the reproductive system is attained only when a girl's growth in height and weight is completed. The pelvis finishes growing even later, not reaching its full size until age 20 or 21. Often teenage mothers give birth to babies who are underweight and have developmental problems because the mothers have not completed their own growth.

Adolescent Changes in Body Composition

Most medical textbooks describe the changes in girls' body size and in their reproductive systems as well as the hormonal changes that take place during adolescence. But a fundamental aspect of growing up that is *not* usually described, as I learned, is a change in the girls' body composition—the relative weight of water, protein (muscle and organ), bone, and fat inside their bodies. These changes accelerate during the adolescent growth spurt, and that was what I wanted to know more about, especially about the changes in body fat.

Of course, the question then arose, How do you measure body fat in a live body? Obviously, you cannot cut people up and measure their body fat. At the time I was researching body composition, there were only indirect methods. Now, we have magnetic resonance imaging (MRI) and other methods that do not involve radiation, so we can safely scan the fat "depots" in the body to determine body fat accurately. We did use MRI later, as I describe in chapter 7, but not until more than ten years after I began investigating body composition.

At the time, the best indirect method of measuring body fat was to measure the total amount of water in the body. Unlike the lean body mass (muscle, organs, and bone), fat contains very little water, so knowing the body's total water content helps indicate the amount of body fat a person has. The fatter you are, the lower the amount of water in your body as a percentage of your weight; the leaner you are, the greater the amount of water as a percentage of your weight.

DRYING OUT AS YOU AGE

As you age, the percentage of water in your body goes down and the percentage of fat goes up (see figure 7 below). Women and men "dry out" as they age because, in a well-fed society like ours, they became fatter. Also, as discussed in chapter 1, women have double the amount of body fat compared to men when they are grown up, so they have a lower percentage of body water (50 percent) than men do (60 percent).

WHAT ARE YOU WEIGHING?

One way to think about body composition—a complicated subject, as I discovered when I became interested in determining fatness in a quantitative way—is to think about what you are weighing when you step on the scale. One thing you are weighing is the water in your body; if you are an adult female, water is half of your body weight. In both men and women, most of the water is in the lean body mass. In fact, 72 percent of the lean body mass is water; surprisingly this percentage is constant among adult animals as well as humans.

It is gruesome, but by actual measurement from autopsies,

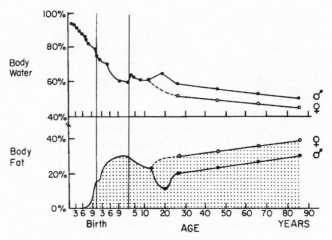

Figure 7. Percentages of body water and fat in men and women from birth to age 85. The percentage of body weight represented by fat increases in females after age 10, during the adolescent growth spurt, and increases in males considerably later, after completion of growth in height and weight. At the same time, the percentage of body weight represented by water decreases because fat has little water compared with the muscles and other parts of the lean body mass (the skeleton and body organs). The body water percentage is therefore an index of fatness. By age 18, when growth is complete, well-nourished U.S. women are typically about 26–28 percent fat; men are about 12–14 percent fat. Adapted from B. Friis-Hansen, "Hydrometry of Growth and Aging," in *Human Body Composition,* Symposia of the Society for the Study of Human Biology, vol. 7, ed. Josef Brožek (Oxford: Pergamon Press, 1965), 191–209.

when you weigh a *fat-free,* normal adult body (male or female), then dry it in an oven, the amount of water lost in the drying averages 72 percent of the original weight. Note that I specified *adult* lean body mass. Children have a higher percentage of water in their lean body mass because they have a smaller proportion of skeleton, which has the lowest percentage of water. As children become taller and have a greater proportion of bone, the percentage of water in their lean body mass begins to fall to 72 percent.

ESTIMATING BODY FAT FROM BODY WATER

Each of the tissues and organs in the body has a different percentage of water, as shown in the table below.

Organ/Tissue	Percentage of Water
Skeletal muscle	79
Heart	83
Skin (fat free)	69
Liver	71
Brain	77
Kidney	81
Skeleton	36

Note that the brain is 77 percent water. Mind-boggling!

Since the water in the lean body mass always totals about 72 percent (because of the differing proportions in the adult body of the tissues listed above), if you measure the total body water of a woman or man and divide it by 0.72, you will get a number for the lean body mass:

$$\frac{\text{Total body water (liters)}}{0.72} = \text{lean body mass (kilograms)}$$

Then, when you subtract the lean body mass from body weight, you obtain the amount of fat, as shown below.

Body weight (kg) − lean body mass (kg) = fat (kg)

(A kilogram is equal to 2.2 pounds. To convert kilograms to pounds, multiply by 2.2.)

You can measure the amount of water in the body directly; it is not difficult or complicated.[1] We measured the body

1. A person drinks a small amount of "heavy water," or deuterium oxide. Deuterium is a stable isotope of hydrogen. It is heavier than the ordinary hydrogen atom because it has a neutron in its nucleus; it has an atomic weight of two. Ordinary hydrogen has only a proton in its nucleus; it has an atomic weight of one. Deuterium can be detected by small differences in the weight. You can give a known amount of the heavy water (e.g., 2 oz or 50 g), and wait for it to be distributed through the general body fluids, which takes two or three hours. Then you draw a known amount of blood plasma and analyze it for how much heavy water it contains, by infrared spectropho-

water of the athletes when we studied the disruption of the menstrual cycle described in chapter 8.

WHY BODY WATER MATTERS

Knowing a person's total body water is useful medically. If you were to go into shock, for example, doctors would need to know immediately how much fluid and electrolytes to give you. They could not stop to measure your body water directly, so they would estimate it from your age, sex, height, and weight, using equations derived from direct measurements of healthy normal subjects. I used these equations to find how a girl's body composition changes as she matures sexually. Fortunately for me, the most significant research on changes in body water of men and women as they age was done in Boston by Dr. Francis Moore, then the chief of surgery of Peter Bent Brigham Hospital, and his co-investigators; together they published *The Body Cell Mass,* a very important work on human body composition.

A FATNESS INDICATOR

I latched onto *total water as percentage of body weight*—an index of fatness—after reading a monograph by a Danish physician, Dr. B. Friis-Hansen, who had worked with Dr. Moore. Dr. Friis-Hansen measured changes in body water for men and women directly from birth to adulthood (see figure 7 earlier in this chapter). In his monograph, Dr. Friis-Hansen observed that while the *absolute* amount of body water is important, he found clinically that *total water as a percentage of body weight* was even more important because it was a fatness index.

Therefore, the first things I wanted to know about the 181 girls I was studying were the changes in body water, lean

---

tometry. From the amount of the dilution of the sample you gave, you can calculate the total amount of water in which the heavy water was diluted. Body water measurements are usually made in a hospital or clinic.

body mass, and fat up to menarche, and then the total water as a percentage of body weight for each girl *at menarche*. It was easy to do because I knew each girl's height and weight during the spurt and at menarche. I used each girl's data to find out how a girl's body composition changes as she matures sexually to menarche.

Learning about changes in body composition from the changes in body water gave me new insight into the growth spurt. Both early- and late-maturing girls had a huge increase in body fat, from 11 pounds (5 kg) at the beginning of the spurt to 24 pounds (11 kg) at menarche, an increase of 120 percent. Their lean body mass increased by only about 44 percent. Thus, I learned that during the spurt the ratio of lean body mass to fat changed—from 5 to 1 at the start of the spurt to 3 to 1 by the time of menarche.

RELATIVE FATNESS

Now I asked the question, What did the shortest, lightest girls at menarche have in common with the tallest, heaviest girls at menarche? Their *relative fatness*, indicated by their total water as a percentage of body weight, was the answer. When girls had menarche, whether early or late, their total water was about 55 percent of body weight, which meant that 22 percent of their body weight was fat! I could hardly believe it. But I confirmed this high percentage by consulting the few other studies in which body water had been measured directly in normal girls in the age range of menarche.

I remember my excitement when I calculated that relative fatness result, because I thought that I might be able to *predict* menarche from the index of fatness. At the time my colleague, Roger Revelle, was attending at a conference at the nearby Massachusetts Institute of Technology. I rushed down to tell him the latest result. He was excited, too.

One other piece of evidence focused my attention on relative fatness. When I followed girls individually through the adolescent growth spurt to menarche, I found they remained in the same percentiles of relative fatness (that is, the plumper

girls remained together and the leaner girls remained together) all the way through the spurt to menarche, whereas
they did not remain in the same percentiles of height or body
weight.

In addition, I found that something that is true for all domestic animals is also true for early- and late-maturing girls.
As girls grow during the spurt, body fat increases at a faster
rate with increasing lean body mass in fast-growing early
maturers than it does in slower-growing late maturers. This
explains why early maturers have more fat on average at
menarche than do late maturers, even though both groups
have the same lean body mass.

This effect creates a problem for animal breeders. The
public wants lean beef, lamb, and pork, but animal breeders
want their animals to grow up quickly. You can see the
dilemma: animals that grow up quickly make more fat per
unit of lean body mass. The effect is a happy one, however,
for girls: a slower rate of growth from leaner diets, with less
fat, makes for a leaner body composition up to menarche and
in later years, benefiting long-term health.

PREDICTING MENARCHE FOR ANORECTIC GIRLS

Now that I had an index of fatness (total water as a percentage of body weight) for 181 normal girls at menarche, was it
possible to predict menarche for a prepubertal girl? To determine this I needed a group of girls with accurate height and
weight measurements and an accurate history of whether
they had had menarche. Girls with anorexia nervosa were
just the kind of subject I was looking for. Also, studying such
girls could be helpful in learning more about anorexia nervosa, a psychogenic disease that involves more than just excessive dieting.

Typically, anorectic girls are adolescents 12 to 16 years
old; most have not had menarche. They lose a lot of weight
by starving themselves and by exercising excessively; they
usually weigh 30 percent less than the normal weight for

their height. They often look like living skeletons, yet they deny their thinness. They look in the mirror and say to themselves, "I am overweight; I am too fat." They often refuse to eat altogether, even when their lives are threatened. Anorectics have a morbid fear of eating fat; I learned, for example, that some girls blotted butter off toast. As has been known since the mid-nineteenth century, their drastic dieting and excessive exercise, which results in extreme weight loss, delay menarche or stop their menstrual cycles. In fact, some psychiatrists think that one of the motivations of anorectic girls in losing so much weight is to "turn off" their sexuality.

Since anorexia nervosa can be life threatening, girls who become too thin are hospitalized and treated to encourage eating and regaining weight into the normal range. When these girls have gained sufficient weight, their vital signs, pulse rate, thyroid metabolism, and other metabolic indicators return to normal, and they are allowed to leave the hospital.

I wanted to know the weight and height of each girl upon discharge from the hospital, her relative fatness, and when she started or resumed normal menstrual cycles. A psychiatrist at Children's Hospital in Boston, Dr. Eugene Piazza, was interested in collaborating on such a study, so I examined the girls' medical records to collect the data.

Consulting with Robert Reed, a biostatistician and an authority on adolescent growth at the Harvard School of Public Health, we found that the easiest way to compare the anorectic girls with the normal girls we had already studied was to draw a grid of heights and weights, as shown in figure 8 below. The diagonal lines are the percentiles of total water as percentage of body weight, or fatness index, at menarche of the normal girls I had studied. Girls in the average (50th) percentile, represented by the middle line, had total water equaling 55 percent of body weight, equivalent to 22 percent body fat. The leanest girls, who were in the 10th percentile, had total water of 59.8 percent (equivalent to 17 percent fat); the plumpest girls, in the 90th percentile, had total water of 50.2 percent (equivalent to 30 percent fat).

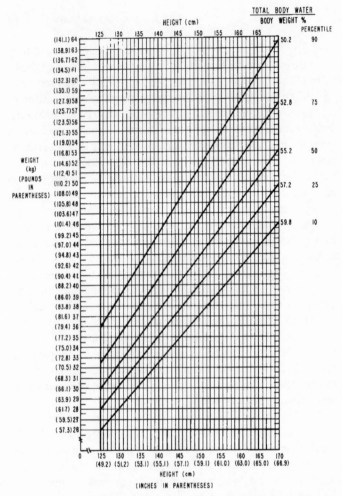

Figure 8. The minimum weight necessary at a particular height for the onset of menstrual cycles (menarche), indicated on the weight scale by the 10th percentile diagonal line of total water/body weight percent (59.8 percent) as it crosses the vertical height lines. See example of 15-year-old girl in text. *Height growth of girls must be completed or approaching completion at this time.* Only the *minimum* weight can be predicted for a particular height. The minimum weight for height for menarche is equivalent to 17 percent fat of body weight. From R. E. Frisch and J. W. McArthur, "Menstrual Cycles: Fatness as a Determinant of Minimum Weight for Height Necessary for Their Maintenance or Onset," *Science* 185 (1973): 949. Copyright © 1973 by the American Association for the Advancement of Science. Reprinted with permission of the American Association for the Advancement of Science.

Minimum Weights for Menarche

Then, I checked the anorectic girls' medical records to find out at what weight for her height each girl had stopped her cycles if she had had them, or what her weight was if she had not had menarche. I learned that no girl had menstrual cycles if she was below a minimum weight for her height as indicated by the fatness index of 59.8 percent total body water, the 10th percentile of normal girls at menarche. (It is the bottom diagonal line in the diagram.) This may seem very technical, but actually it is easy to read off the minimum weight for each girl: find her height along the bottom of the diagram, then proceed up until you reach the first diagonal line, and then check the vertical axis on the left for the corresponding weight. For example, a girl who is 63 inches (160 cm) tall must weigh *at least* 90 pounds (41 kg) before menstrual cycles would be expected to begin.

After the anorectic girls were discharged from the hospital, they reported periodically to Dr. Piazza. Most were *at* the minimum weight for their height. I wanted to know if and when they gained weight and whether their menstrual cycles started or resumed. I was amazed to find that most girls remained at their minimum weight for height and had no menstrual cycles. The few girls who exceeded the minimum weight for their height either had menarche or resumed menstrual cycles.

Minimum Weight for Maintenance of Cycles at Age 16 to 18 and Over

I was curious about older women over 18 who indulged in what their doctors called "injudicious dieting" to remain slim as models. Did they fit the minimum weight-for-height predictions that applied to anorectic girls, most of whom were in their early teens? No, they did not. It was back to the drawing board.

I then tracked the changes in weight and fatness for each normal girl, starting at menarche and continuing until she

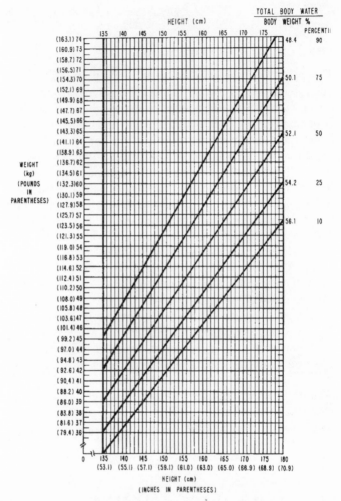

Figure 9. The minimum weight necessary at a particular height for the restoration and maintenance of menstrual cycles, indicated on the weight scale by the 10th percentile line of total water/body weight percent (56.1 percent) as it crosses the vertical height line. See example of 20-year-old woman in text. From R. E. Frisch and J. W. McArthur, "Menstrual Cycles: Fatness as a Determinant of Minimum Weight for Height Necessary for Their Maintenance or Onset," *Science* 185 (1973): 949. Copyright © 1973 by the American Association for the Advancement of Science. Reprinted with permission of the American Association for the Advancement of Science.

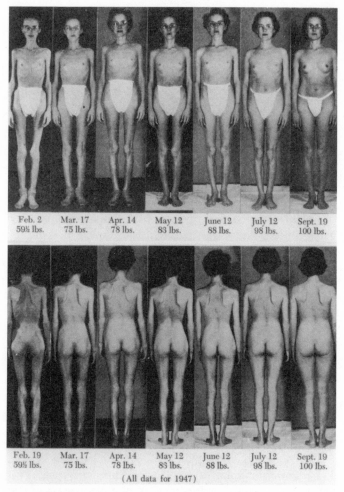

| Feb. 2 | Mar. 17 | Apr. 14 | May 12 | June 12 | July 12 | Sept. 19 |
| 59½ lbs. | 75 lbs. | 78 lbs. | 83 lbs. | 88 lbs. | 98 lbs. | 100 lbs. |

| Feb. 19 | Mar. 17 | Apr. 14 | May 12 | June 12 | July 12 | Sept. 19 |
| 59½ lbs. | 75 lbs. | 78 lbs. | 83 lbs. | 88 lbs. | 98 lbs. | 100 lbs. |

(All data for 1947)

Figure 10. A 32-year-old woman's recovery from anorexia nervosa, a disease she had suffered from since the age of 18. When admitted to a clinic she was 62.5 inches tall (158.8 cm) and weighed 59.6 pounds (27 kg). With successive weight gain, she attained 100 pounds, the minimum weight for her height (as predicted by the fatness index discussed earlier in this chapter) for resumption or maintenance of menstrual cycles. Note that at 100 pounds she is no longer gaunt. From A. Keys et al., *The Biology of Human Starvation*, vol. 1 (Minneapolis: University of Minnesota Press, 1950), 100. Copyright © 1950 by the University of Minnesota. Reprinted with permission of the University of Minnesota Press.

finished growing at 18. There was the answer: the girls gained another 10 pounds (4.5 kg) of body fat from menarche to the completion of growth; they averaged 26 percent body fat, or 35 pounds (16 kg) of fat! It was hardly believable. At age 18 the average fatness index was 52 percent, and the 10th percentile was 56 percent, equivalent to a *minimum* of 22 percent body fat (see figure 9 above).

I collaborated with Dr. Janet W. McArthur, then a gynecologist at Massachusetts General Hospital, to study the cycles of young women, mostly 18 and older, who dieted and jogged but were not anorectics. They lost a moderate amount of weight, about 10 to 15 percent of their normal weight for height. Using the same technique suggested by Professor Reed, I drew a height–weight grid and placed on the grid the fatness index percentiles (total water as a percentage of body weight) of normal girls at age 18. Then we looked to see who had cycles and who did not. Women who had no cycles fit the new standard very well: for these older women, the fatness index necessary for menstrual cycles was 56.1 percent, the 10th percentile of normal 18-year-old girls *at completion of growth*. Thus, a 20-year-old woman who was 63 inches tall (160 cm) had to weigh at least 101 pounds (46 kg) before menstrual cycles would be expected to resume (see figure 10 below). The minimum weights for height for the onset or maintenance of regular cycles are listed in the table at the end of the chapter.

Dr. McArthur and I published our results in *Science* in 1974. These minimum "turn off" and "turn on" weights for the onset or maintenance of menstrual cycles are now used clinically. They are used as target, or threshold, weights for United States and European women who have no cycles because they are too thin from constant dieting or intensive exercise or both.

Note that we could predict only the *minimum* weight for a particular height at which cycles would occur. We could not predict *above* the minimum weight for these women, or for the younger girls at menarche. Note also that the minimum weight for height was predicted from total water as percentage of body weight, not from *fat* as percentage of body weight (although the water percentage is *equivalent* to a particular fat percentage).[2] This suggests the importance of the ratio of lean body mass to fat: normally it is about 3 to 1 at menarche and 2.5 to 1 at the completion of growth at age 18. For example, a newborn is about 16 percent body fat, close to the equivalent minimum fat percentage for menarche, but the infant's lean body mass is obviously not in the adolescent size range. In contrast, by the end of the growth spurt, a girl attains close to an adult-size lean body mass, accompanied by a large increase in body fat.

Of course, young women who have no cycles or irregular ones need to be checked for pathologies of the reproductive system. But now, if physicians find nothing wrong or abnormal, the women's weight for height can be checked. Usually, these women are about eight to ten pounds below the minimum weight necessary for their height. Many decide to have a baby after the age of 30, and because fecundity (the ability to conceive) begins to decrease after age 35, they find that conceiving becomes difficult, even after surpassing the minimum weight. To my surprise, a number of women told me they were unwilling or unable to gain the pounds necessary to exceed the minimum weight. When asked why, they often replied, "I don't feel right being so heavy." That body weight isn't "so heavy" at all, of course, so what it is they are feeling when they are over the threshold weight as opposed to below it is not known.

2. There's been some confusion about the fact that you cannot predict the minimum weights from fat as percent of body weight, even though the minimum weights represent a fat percentage. The reason *total water as percent of body weight* is the predictor is that absolute amount of body water (liters) tells you how much lean body mass you have (your muscles, internal organs, and bone), and the size of that lean body mass indicates whether you are "grown up" or not. The *percentage* of body water tells you how much fat you have in relation to the lean body mass. Thus, you can think of attaining reproductive maturity as growing up to the amount of lean body mass necessary to produce a viable infant, that is, growing up into the normal adult size range, and them glomming on the necessary amount of fat for the energy to be a successful reproducer.

Precautions on the Use
of the Minimum Weights

The standards discussed above apply as yet only to Caucasian American and European females. Different ethnic groups and races have different average weights at menarche, and it is not yet known whether the different weights represent the same critical body composition of relative fatness. We know, for example, that the average weight at menarche of Japanese girls is 97 pounds (44 kg), but we do not know what that weight represents in body composition.

Other factors, such as emotional stress, can affect the onset or maintenance of menstrual cycles. In these cases, menstrual cycles may cease without weight loss and sometimes may not resume even if the minimum weight for height has been achieved or exceeded. Before determining whether undernutrition or intensive exercise is involved in the delay of menarche (i.e., after age 16 in nonathletic girls) or in irregular or absent cycles, it is important to rule out any other contributing factors.

Very muscular athletes such as Olympic oarswomen or body builders whose weight may be normal for their height may still lack menstrual cycles because they have a low percentage of body fat. (Muscles are heavy.) We know that if these women exercise less and increase their caloric intake, cycles usually start or resume, but we cannot predict the weight for height at which this will happen. Often there is no change in weight as fat replaces muscle.

When the minimum weights were first used clinically, some doctors did not yet connect body fat and fertility. I still remember, twenty years later, the look of utter incredulity on the face of a Nobel Laureate scientist who asked me what I would be speaking on at an endocrine conference. When I replied, "body fat, menarche, and ovulation," he was speechless. It was as if I had said something totally irrelevant, like "Girls are sugar and spice and all things nice." I'm glad to say that my audience at the conference, including the Nobel Lau-

MINIMUM WEIGHT FOR PARTICULAR HEIGHT NECESSARY FOR THE
ONSET OR RESTORATION OF MENSTRUAL CYCLES

	Menarche or Primary Amenorrhea		Secondary Amenorrhea	
Height (in.)	Minimum Weight (lb.)[a] (10th percentile)	Average Weight (lb.) (50th percentile)	Minimum Weight (lb.)[b] (10th percentile)	Average Weight (lb.) (50th percentile)
53.1	66.7	76.8	74.6	85.6
53.9	68.6	79.2	76.8	88.2
54.7	70.6	81.4	79.0	90.6
55.5	72.6	83.6	81.2	93.3
56.3	74.4	85.8	83.4	95.7
57.1	76.3	88.2	85.6	98.3
57.9	78.3	90.4	87.8	100.8
58.7	80.3	92.6	90.0	103.4
59.4	82.3	94.8	92.2	105.8
60.2	84.3	97.2	94.4	108.5
61.0	86.2	99.4	96.6	110.9
61.8	88.2	101.6	98.8	113.3
62.6	90.2	103.8	101.0	115.9
63.4	92.2	106.3	103.2	118.4
64.2	93.9	108.5	105.4	121.0
65.0	95.9	110.7	107.6	123.4
65.7	97.9	113.1	109.8	126.1
66.5	99.9	115.3	112.0	128.5
67.3	101.9	117.5	114.0	131.1
68.1	103.8	119.7	116.2	133.5
68.9	105.8	122.1	118.4	136.0
69.7	107.8	124.3	120.6	138.6
70.5	109.6	126.5	122.8	141.0
71.3	111.8	128.7	125.2	143.7

Source: Data from R. E. Frisch and J. W. McArthur, "Menstrual Cycles: Fatness as a Determinant of Minimum Weight for Height Necessary for Their Maintenance or Onset," *Science* 185 (1974): 949–51, figs. 1 and 2.

[a]Equivalent to 17 percent fat/body weight; height growth must be completed or nearing completion.

[b]Equivalent to 22 percent fat/body weight.

reate, found my talk on the role of body fat interesting and provocative; as they say in the trade, it was well received.

I was invited to speak at that small, elegant endocrine conference in Venice by the recommendation of a very distinguished endocrinologist whom I regarded as a mentor, Seymour Reichlin, then chief of endocrinology at Tufts Medical School and president of the Endocrine Society (now emeritus at the University of Arizona, Tucson). I met Dr. Reichlin when I was studying metabolic rates—a very difficult, often murky subject. His chapter in the book I was reading was so beautifully clear that I called Harvard's Countway Library of Medicine to find out where he was working so that I could meet him. To my great pleasure, he had just moved to Boston. Dr. Reichlin, as I learned, held a Ph.D. in addition to an M.D., and he had worked with Cambridge scientist Geoffrey Harris in England, the discoverer of the hypothalamic control of reproduction. Dr. Reichlin thought my critical fatness hypothesis an interesting path of research and encouraged me to continue. Over the years, his criticisms and comments have been invaluable.

7   Pubertal Body Fat—Sex Fat?

A Neat Mechanism for
Reproductive Success

That something so small—and so crude—as a five-pound weight loss or gain around the threshold weight can turn menstrual cycles on or off may seem improbable in this age of molecular biology. But much research has shown that such relatively small decreases (or increases) in weight are accompanied by a fall (or rise) of the hormones necessary for cycles and ovulation to occur.

As I explained in chapter 4, the hypothalamus secretes gonadotropin-releasing hormone (GnRH), a controlling hormone in reproduction. In a normal, mature woman, GnRH signals "go" to the pituitary-ovary axis, but in too thin or too lean women, GnRH is secreted in an abnormal pattern. Due to the hypothalamic dysfunction, the normal cascade of pituitary hormones—luteinizing hormone (LH), follicle-stimulating hormone (FSH), and estrogen—is turned off, and such women do not ovulate or menstruate. Moreover, LH secretion and the response of the pituitary gland to GnRH are reduced in direct correlation with the amount of weight loss. In addition, the twenty-four-hour pattern of LH secretion resembles that of prepubertal or early pubertal children, who have differences in night and day secretion. Weight gain restores the normal postmenarcheal pattern of secretion (see figure 11 below).

There is further evidence of the link between hypothala-

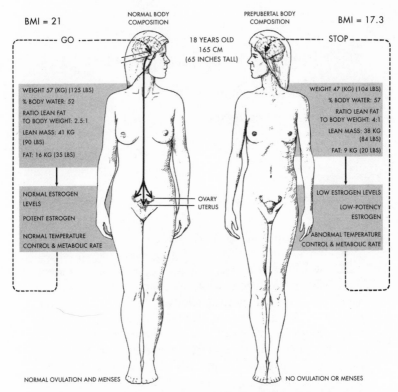

Figure 11. A woman of normal weight for her height (left) who loses about 15 percent of her body weight (right) may not appear to be shockingly thin. But she will have lost about one-third of her body fat and may stop menstruating because hypothalamic functioning, which controls reproductive ability, has become abnormal. Drawing by Carol Donner; reprinted with permission of Carol Donner. From R. E. Frisch, "Fatness and Fertility," *Scientific American* 258 (1988): 88.

mic control and fatness. Underweight women who are injected with GnRH respond with a pattern of secretion of FSH and LH similar to that of prepubertal children: the FSH is greater than the LH response. The return of normal LH responsiveness is correlated with weight gain. When these underweight women gain enough weight to enter the normal range for their height, the pulsatile secretion of GnRH attains the adult pattern, and the cascade of hormones it stimulates then reaches the normal range as well, thus stimulating the growth of a follicle and ovulation. In my view, this type of turn-off by the hypothalamus is adaptive: the brain says no, turning off the pituitary hormones, because underweight women do not have the relative fatness necessary to have a viable infant; they are at high risk of giving birth to an infant who is too lightweight to survive.

OTHER LINKAGES OF BODY FAT AND REPRODUCTIVE ABILITY

Even before the evidence of GnRH control by the brain was known and leptin was discovered, scientists learned that body fat could directly affect reproductive ability in four ways. Most important was the unexpected finding by Pentti Siiteri and Paul MacDonald in 1973 that a body tissue—fat—can be a source of estrogen even though it is not a hormonal gland. Many researchers then showed that specific depots of body fat in the body could convert androgens, a male hormone, to estrogen through the action of the enzyme aromatase. Fat of the breast, fat of the abdomen, and fat of the omentum (the large, fatty apron that covers the internal organs in the abdomen) all make estrogen.

My collaborators and I found that the fatty marrow of the long bones also makes estrogen. Most bones have red marrow, which is the source of red blood cells and many of the other blood cells circulating in the body. But at puberty, most of the red marrow in the long bones of the arms and legs is replaced with fatty marrow. This happens in both girls and boys.

I became intrigued with fatty marrow after hearing a lecture given by Harvard professor Judah Folkman on the development of blood vessels (angiogenesis). Dr. Folkman described how the cartilage at the ends of the long bones could not be penetrated by blood vessels; there was some kind of inhibition. These growing points of cartilage, called epiphyses, become bone when growth ends after the adolescent growth spurt. That is also the time when long bones become filled with fatty marrow. Since I knew fat could make estrogen, I wondered if the fatty marrow of the long bones made estrogen from androgens. One could speculate that the estrogen made in the marrow reverses the inhibition of blood vessels in the cartilage of the epiphyses, allowing the epiphyses to "close" with the formation of bone.

How might I obtain live marrow to test whether it makes estrogen? As I found out, one way is to contact an orthopedic surgeon who does hip replacements. After filling out many papers and obtaining permission, I arranged to be at the hospital during the operation. Eventually, a nurse appeared at the operating room door with a small vial. I put the vial into ice, then rushed to the Laboratory of Human Reproduction to meet my biochemical collaborator, Dr. Jack Canick, who had all the necessary solutions ready. We did that for six different patients. All the fatty marrows were found to convert androgens to estrogen, and we reported our results in 1980 in the *Journal of Clinical Endocrinology and Metabolism*.

SPIDERY ARMS AND LEGS OF BALLET DANCERS

What happens if there isn't enough estrogen in general (not necessarily from marrow) to close the epiphyses? If you have seen a ballet company, you have probably noticed that most of the dancers look like spiders because of their very long arms and legs. That is because most ballet dancers start their training before menarche, and they stay skinny. Therefore, estrogen levels do not increase, and the dancers' arms and legs keep growing. You may also notice that many dancers are flat-chested; that is because the breasts don't develop without an increase in estrogen. Athletes who begin their training before menarche often show the same overly long arms and legs. Normally, adult height is equal to the length of arm span. Many of the female (and male) athletes we measured had arm spans two or three inches longer than their height.

POTENT AND NONPOTENT FORMS OF ESTROGEN

A second, very important way that body fat influences reproductive ability is the effect of body weight, hence fatness, on the metabolism of estrogen. In 1975 Jack Fishman, Leon Bradlow, and their collaborators then at Rockefeller University in New York found that very lean women made more of a nonpotent form of estrogen than did normal women. This nonpotent form does not stimulate the cells of the lining of the uterus to divide and prepare for the implantation of an embryo, and it does not stimulate the cells of the breast to divide and grow milk-producing ducts.

With a high proportion of the body's estrogen metabolized to this form, the entire reproductive system shifts to a nonreproductive phase. It is as if the system were put on idle while waiting for more propitious times to gear up again. The change in the ratio of the nonpotent form to the potent form can be a partial one, so that a woman is still fertile but exposed to relatively lower levels of potent estrogen. This may explain the lower lifetime occurrence of cancers of the breast and reproductive system we observed among former college athletes compared to their sedentary classmates (see chapter 9).

Fishman and Bradlow have shown that in lean women, a special enzyme in the liver brings about an increase in nonpotent estrogen. My colleagues and I have confirmed that in lean athletes, nonpotent estrogen increases as body fat, measured with magnetic resonance imaging (MRI), decreases.

ENVIRONMENTAL FACTORS: SMOKING, CABBAGES, AND A LOW-FAT DIET

What cues the enzyme to metabolize estrogen in the potent form or the nonpotent form? That is still not known; what is known is that ordinary environmental factors affect the ratio of potent to nonpotent estrogen. Smoking, for example, causes an increase in the nonpotent form, which explains why smokers have a lower incidence of ovarian cancer. No one, however, recommends smoking for this or any other reason; the risk of lung cancer is so much higher in smokers.

What you eat can also affect the metabolism of estrogen. Vegetables of the cabbage family (including broccoli and brussels sprouts) contain substances called indoles that increase the proportion of nonpotent estrogen. This may be one reason for the lower incidence of breast cancer among women in developing countries where lots of cabbage-type vegetables are consumed. A low-fat diet also raises the proportion of nonpotent estrogen. Though it is still considered controversial, there is a lot of evidence that a low-fat diet reduces the risk of breast cancer; the shift of the ratio in favor of the nonpotent form of estrogen may be one mechanism that lowers the risk.

In contrast to lean women, obese women metabolize less of the nonpotent form of estrogen and have a relative increase in the potent form. Obese women are at higher risk for cancer of the breast and the endometrium. Again, one of the factors may be the relative increase in the potent form of estrogen.

Sex-Hormone-Binding Globulin

The third way that the amount of fat changes the body's hormonal environment is by affecting the ability of estrogen to bind to a special protein called sex-hormone-binding globulin. Estrogens attach to this protein; when they are attached, they have no physiological effect and become inactive. In obese women and in early-maturing young girls, who are relatively fatter than later maturers, estrogen has a decreased ability to bind to the sex-hormone-binding globulin. That means there is more free estrogen circulating in the body. Sex-hormone-binding globulin thus regulates the availability of estrogen to the brain and to many other target tissues such as the breast and uterus. Changes in the proportion of body fat can affect both fertility and the risk of reproductive-system cancers.

Adipose tissue stores steroid hormones; this may be one

more way by which body fat affects reproductive ability, but very little is known about how the release of these hormones affects reproduction. We do know that the fat in the breast influences the estrogen levels locally, which may be a factor in the risk of breast cancer.

DISTURBANCES IN THE REGULATION OF BODY TEMPERATURE

Finally, changes in relative fatness may affect reproductive ability indirectly by inducing disturbances in the hypothalamic regulation of body temperature and energy balance. Very lean women, both athletes and nonathletes, do not regulate their temperature normally. They are usually hypothermic—their body temperature is below the normal temperature of 98.6°F. In fact, when we were studying runners and swimmers, we often heard athletes say, "My temperature is up to 98.6—I must have the flu." Studies of women with moderate weight loss, in the range of 10 to 15 percent below normal, showed that these underweight, nonathletic women could not control their temperature when they were placed in a too hot or too cold environment.

In my view, this may be a good reason for the hypothalamus to turn off reproductive ability. A pregnant woman should be in a steady state while growing a baby; her temperature should not fluctuate up and down. Whatever the reason, lean women who cannot control their temperature have a delayed response or lack of response to GnRH, the controlling reproductive hormone; thus their fertility is turned off.

And now there is leptin, a direct connection from body fat to the hypothalamus. It takes a whole chapter (10) to describe the importance of leptin.

THE FATNESS–FERTILITY CONNECTION

I think it is a neat connection: body fat links how much you eat, what kind of food you eat, your level of physical activity, and the environmental temperature with the hypothalamic control of fertility, turning the system on and off. Fat is the most labile (changeable) tissue in the body; therefore, it is a sensitive signaler to the brain—it is the first tissue to recognize and respond to changes in the environment such as food intake and physical activity.

GOING PUBLIC

Until the late 1980s I had published only scientific papers (now more than one hundred) on fatness and fertility. In 1988, the first article I wrote for the general public appeared in *Scientific American,* and I was astounded at the response. I received hundreds of requests for reprints of my article (surely you have guessed the title: "Fatness and Fertility") and many phone calls. One call I still remember was from a man in Hawaii who asked, "Would you please send a reprint and more articles?" When I inquired whether my caller wanted copies of my scientific papers, he replied, "Anything you think will help. We are two runners and we want to have a baby." I even received calls at home. One was from a woman in Adelaide, Australia. My husband answered the phone and said, with some asperity, that I was eating dinner. "Oh, but it's very important," she replied. "I read Dr. Frisch's article, and now I'm pregnant. But my sister is a windsurfer—much too thin. And she wants a baby, too." Could Dr. Frisch please send the *Scientific American* article to her sister? I did. I hope she windsurfed less, ate more, and was successful.

Pierre-Auguste Renoir's "Seated Bather," a beautiful nude, graced the cover of that issue of *Scientific American.* When Ricky Rusting, an admirable editor at *Scientific American,* told me about the cover (which mentioned my article), I objected to the illustration, saying, "Only the science matters, and readers will buy it for the beautiful nude." Ricky assured me that readers would read my article. In any case, it was a best-selling issue, and I'll never know whether it was Renoir's bather or my article that did it.

In 1990, I edited a book called *Adipose Tissue and Reproduction,* published by Karger of Basel, Switzerland. It was the first scientific book to focus on the link between adipose tissue (body fat) and reproduction. I especially enjoyed writing the introductory chapter on my "critical fatness" hypothesis and related research because I could include my hypotheses on body fat and fertility and nobody could "blue pencil" them out (which other editors sometimes did to my papers— "too hypothetical," they would comment in the margins).

I contacted a number of experts whose research was relevant to some aspect of the fatness-fertility connection and invited them to contribute chapters to the book. The contributors ranged widely, from biochemists and ecologists to gynecologists and oncologists. I was honored that all these prominent scientists accepted and contributed to the book and Daniel D. Federman, the dean of medical education and professor of medicine at Harvard Medical School, wrote the foreword. (Dr. Federman had an early interest in my research, and I was delighted when I learned he had used my 1988 article in *Scientific American* as a reference in his obstetrics-gynecology course.) *Adipose Tissue and Reproduction* is still in print, and the last time I checked on it at Countway Medical Library, I was very pleased to see that it looked worn from use. It was favorably reviewed in the *New England Journal of Medicine* by another mentor and friend, Dr. Seymour Reichlin, then of Tufts Medical School. My book was published by Karger through the interest of editor Dr. Freddy Homburger, an oncologist who became a close friend and supporter of my ideas. Dr. Homburger was the first to demonstrate that tobacco was carcinogenic.

A FAILURE AND WHAT IT TAUGHT

In the book's preface, I recounted an early experiment by George Corner, an eminent endocrinologist. "A failure and what it taught" is how Dr. Corner described the importance of body size and the efficacy of a hormone. Corner wrote that his fellow researcher, Willard Allen, went off on vacation after they had sent their paper for publication on the effects of extracts of a hormone, progesterone, injected into rabbits.

Corner decided he wanted to repeat the method of preparing the hormone by himself, so he did, and injected the hormone into rabbits, as Allen had done. Nothing happened. By the time Allen returned, Corner was in a panic; he checked and rechecked his method of preparation; no matter what he did, the rabbits didn't respond. Allen said, "Just show me exactly what you did." After Corner injected the rabbits, Allen said, "Why did you choose the *littler* rabbits? I always preferred the bigger rabbits." The rabbits had a minimum weight; when a rabbit weighed less than 800 grams, there was no response to the hormone. To put it simply, the rabbit wasn't grown up enough to respond to a reproductive hormone that said "go."

In 1998, I received a phone call about body weights and fertility in animals at the other end of the size range—fifty-foot North Atlantic right whales. Marine scientists are worried that the whales are becoming extinct—only about three hundred are left. One of the problems? As I learned from my caller, many females never produce calves. Researchers observed that plankton levels, the whales' main food, are lower. "Poor nutrition and a lack of body fat may have something to do with the whales' reproductive failures," theorized Dr. Michael J. Moore of the Woods Hole Oceanographic Institute. In consequence, they are now measuring the thickness of a whale's blubber (all body fat) with an ultrasonic probe. Adult whales have blubber that is nine and a half inches thick; the blubber of the young calves is half as thick. (Breast milk of a whale is like whipped cream, 50 percent fat, so those calves gain fat quickly under normal circumstances.) Dr. Moore hopes to collect data about blubber thickness in relation to a whale's reproductive history. You can identify a particular whale by its head crest. A whale of an experiment, and right in line with rabbits and the human female.

8 Physical Activity and Too Little Fat

Ballet Dancers, Swimmers, Runners, and Other Athletes

W hen the dancers weigh in," said the voice on the telephone, "the choreographer sits there and watches the scales. If a dancer gains weight, all hell breaks loose." My long-distance caller, back in 1979, was Dr. Lawrence Vincent, a radiologist practicing in New York City. Dr. Vincent primarily treated dancers with physical injuries, usually orthopedic injuries, but he had become interested in their general health problems.

Recalling the 1974 *Science* article on fatness and menstrual cycles that I coauthored with Janet W. McArthur, Dr. Vincent wondered whether I'd like to collaborate with him on a study of the age of menarche and menstrual function of ballet dancers. How had he gotten interested? Walking back and forth from the hospital where he worked, he explained, he often passed students of a nearby ballet company. In his words, "I did not see a starry-eyed ballet student coming from her ballet class; I saw a pale, gaunt seventeen-year-old with dark circles under her eyes and a downcast gaze. Her unhealthy visage bore none of the physical exuberance and vitality usually associated with exercise. She looked terrible." She had danced for seven hours that day and had eaten only an orange and a slice of mango.[1]

1. L. M. Vincent, *Competing with the Sylph: The Quest for the Perfect Dance Body,* 2d ed. (Princeton: Princeton Book Co., 1989), xiv.

As Dr. Vincent found out, the student was typical of most of the dancers; they were obsessed with weight and dieting. What about their reproductive ability? Was it affected, as we would expect it to be, if they were too lean? That is what we would investigate, with the help of the dancers.

BALLET DANCERS WITH REPRODUCTIVE PROBLEMS

One year later, with the collaboration of biostatistician Dr. Grace Wyshak, we reported in the *New England Journal of Medicine* on the reproductive-system problems of young ballet dancers. Of the 89 dancers we studied, 20 had not had menarche even though their age averaged 18.5; of these, 6 were older than 18, and 2 were in their early twenties. Only 29 of the dancers reported regular cycles. Thirteen dancers had no menstrual cycles for more than three months, and 27 reported irregular cycles (intervals between cycles of more than 38 days, but less than three months). Among the dancers who had had menarche, the average age was 13.7, significantly later than the average age (12.6 to 12.8) among the general population. Another researcher studying dancers found the average age of menarche to be 15.

What about their leanness? Dancers who had no cycles or irregular menstrual cycles were leaner than dancers with regular cycles. The 20 dancers reporting "no menarche yet" were the leanest of all. Their body weights were well below the weight for height I could predict from the fatness index as necessary for normal cycles. The 14-year-old girls, for example, reporting "no menarche yet" were the same height, 62 inches (158.7 cm) as nondancing girls at the age of menarche, but they weighed only 92 pounds (42 kg), 13 pounds less on average than well-fed, nondancing girls, whose weight at menarche averaged 105 pounds (47.8 kg).

Two dancers reporting irregular cycles were in the normal range of fatness for maintaining cycles, demonstrating an important exception: that weight is necessary but not sufficient for cycles to occur. Emotional or physical stress may override a normal body weight.

If a dancer had an injury that prevented dancing, and many dancers did, lo and behold, after an interval of time, menarche occurred or cycles resumed if they had stopped. If the dancer became leaner again, menstrual cycles ceased.

After our results were published in 1980 in the *New England Journal of Medicine,* I was amazed at how surprised physicians were at the news. I received many requests for reprints of the article, but by and large, the reaction was astonishment. The dancers' lack of cycles must be explained by something else—maybe only late maturers choose to be ballet dancers. How could things so crude as body weight and the amount of fat and lean mass matter? My reaction was that medical students weren't informed that reproduction had a metabolic cost. As one reproductive endocrinologist explained to me, doctors learn much of their medicine on the wards, and on the wards there are no super lean dancers who had not had menarche or whose menstrual cycles had ceased.

If too lean dancers had menstrual problems, what about too lean athletes? We were lucky that more and more young women were jogging, running competitively, and generally indulging in regular, vigorous exercise. Reports began to appear in the literature that these young women had delayed menarche or problems with their menstrual cycles, correlated with the number of miles they ran per week—the more the miles, the more the menstrual problems.

DECIDING TO STUDY ATHLETES

I was able to study athletes by first trying to study menopause. It sounds improbable, but that's really how it happened. My colleagues and I had submitted a proposal to study the age of menopause of diabetic women. Nothing was known about the topic at the time (about fifteen years ago), and as far as I know, nobody knows about it now. I was interested because it was already being suggested that fatter women have a later age of menopause than do leaner women. I had studied the age of menarche of girls with juvenile-onset diabetes, and they had menarche later than nondiabetic girls because they were leaner than the normal girls. What was the impact of diabetes at the other end of the reproductive life-span?

Unfortunately for my proposed research, nobody in the official agencies was interested in menopause fifteen years ago. In fact, nobody anywhere seemed to be interested in menopausal women. But, I thought, surely there must be somebody. Who? Maybe the manufacturers of Kotex or Tampax? The later the menopause, the more products they would sell. How to contact them?

I settled on Tampax and the direct approach. I found the telephone number of Tampax products and called, asking for the director of the research laboratory. I identified myself to the doctor who answered, saying I was a faculty member of the Department of Population Sciences at the Harvard School of Public Health. "Oh, I know you," he replied. "I'm a consultant to your department." Pleasant as he was, it turned out he didn't care about menopause, either. But, he said, why not study athletes? Maybe he had already heard rumors that some runners and joggers had no menstrual cycles and therefore did not need tampons—a discouraging thought for the manufacturers of Tampax. Maybe he had read our paper on the ballet dancers who reported a high incidence of menstrual problems. Being helpful, he suggested I call the chairman of the Olympic committee; perhaps there would be funds to study women athletes. Much correspondence with the committee followed, and the upshot was that the committee didn't have the money to do a detailed study. Whom to try next?

FINDING AND FUNDING THE ATHLETES

I was very enthusiastic at the suggestion that we study athletes. While I was teaching about moderate weight loss and the absence of menstrual cycles, one of my students had told me, "My roommate is on the crew, and she doesn't have any cycles either when she's in top training." I then prepared a new proposal with Dr. Janet McArthur, then at Massachusetts General Hospital. We were fortunate to be joined by surgeon Tenley Albright, a former Olympic gold medal ice skater, and Drs. Nile Albright and Hollis Albright, all directors of the Advanced Medical Research Foundation of Boston, which sponsored the study.

What did we want to find out? Well, for one thing, would the athletes show the same correlation of leanness and menstrual problems as the ballet dancers did? After we reported in the *New England Journal of Medicine* that ballet dancers had a later average age of menarche than nondancers, other investigators found the same delay for athletes. But instead of reasoning that something about the exercise, if it had begun before menarche, might have delayed menarche, a common explanation was that all the girls who decided to become athletes were late maturers. If only late maturers wanted to be athletes, of course the average age of the athletes would be later than the general population. That explanation was also offered for the dancers. This solution presumed that all the early maturers hated exercise and were lolling on sofas eating jelly doughnuts. There was no evidence for this explanation, but it was popular nonetheless.

To gather some evidence on the question, we planned to ask the runners and swimmers in our study how old they were when they began regular exercise, how intense the exercise was, and their age of menarche as precisely as possible in years and months. We also wanted to know their medical history and whether their menstrual cycles, if they had them, were regular or irregular. We told them how to classify their menstrual periodicity: "primary amenorrhea" meant that menarche had not yet occurred (the athletes were 17 and older); "secondary amenorrhea" meant that cycles occurred at least six months apart. Irregular cycles differed in length by nine or more days.

To recruit athletes for the study, we put up notices in the Harvard athletic centers and advertised in the *Harvard Crimson* for undergraduate control subjects. Athletes are very interested in what's going on in their bodies and were glad to comply with our requests. We took physical measurements and questioned them about their diet and the regularity of their menstrual cycles (many who had irregular cycles were relieved to find that they weren't alone). It was easy to recruit control subjects who weren't exercising: it was becoming fashionable to be body conscious, and the control subjects were measured just as the athletes were. We recruited 21 team swimmers, 17 runners, and 10 controls. We saw them regularly to collect the data, and we grew to love them all.

Our study was a prospective study, meaning that we had baseline information on each of the subjects: height, weight, age of menarche, pulse rate, thigh measurements, estimated relative fatness, menstrual periodicity if any—all the characteristics that we thought would help us describe how athletes differed from control subjects during training. Then, we followed each athlete and control subject through the training season, instructing them to keep a record of each menstrual cycle in detail, recording the first and last day of each period and the characteristics of the bleeding. Each study participant was given an oral basal-temperature thermometer to record her bedtime temperature (and the time it was taken) each day. Evening temperatures were used because temperature fluctuations are fewer at night. By plotting these temperatures, we could determine whether ovulation had taken place during a monthly cycle and also check out reports of menstrual periodicity.

One of our simpler measurements was that of breast size. Breast size was very difficult to measure, so we just asked the size of the breast cup of the brassiere each participant wore. In those days, about fifteen years ago, young women still wore a brassiere with an A, B, C, or D cup size. We soon learned that the swimmers who reported a C or D cup size were recreational swimmers; they had never made a team. There were no runners with C or D cup size. Soon, to our dismay, the one-size brassiere arrived, and then a lot of the young women stopped wearing brassieres at all, so we had to give up on breast size.

Ten years later when we studied runners and swimmers again, we measured fatness by using magnetic resonance imaging (MRI), which is noninvasive and gives no radiation dose. With MRI, we could quantify both subcutaneous and internal fat at the level of the breast. Let me jump ahead to say that much to the chagrin of the athletes, this was the site where they lost the most fat rather than at the hips and thighs, where they wanted to lose it.

The baseline temperature measurements of most of the well-trained athletes amazed us right from the start. Their evening temperatures ranged around 96.5°F. Practically no one had an evening temperature of 98.6°F except the C and D cup recreational swimmers. If anyone recorded 98°F or so, they would note that they "had the flu."

ATHLETIC TRAINING DELAYED MENARCHE

As with the ballet dancers we studied, the average age of menarche for the athletes (13.9) was significantly older than the average age for the general population (12.8) and for the control subjects (12.7). Nothing new. But if you added up the menarcheal ages of the eighteen athletes who started their training *before* they had menarche, the average menarcheal age was 15.1, whereas for the twenty athletes who started training after menarche, the age was 12.9—similar to that of the control subjects and the general population. So it wasn't true that all athletes were genetically late maturers. It mattered whether you started your training before or after menarche—something about the training itself delayed menarche. Among this group of athletes, menarche was delayed five months for each year of training—a big effect.

Some of the athletes were 19, 20, or 21 years old and had never had a menstrual cycle. They were usually California girls who had joined teams at a young age and trained year-round. Some of these early-starter athletes had been taken to a doctor by an anxious mother who wanted to know why her daughter was different from everyone else in her class and hadn't had menarche yet. Usually, the doctor found nothing wrong, and those who read the current literature told the mothers to wait until their daughters stopped being so athletic. But some mothers insisted that their daughters have cycles, so the young women were put on estrogen to simulate the normal process. Most of these young women quietly went off the hormone regimen because they felt better without it, and as we learned from the ballet dancers, normal periods began when they stopped exercising or reduced the intensity of training.

At the beginning of the training season, athletes who had first started training before menarche reported a higher number of irregular and missed cycles than did those who started training after menarche. During the athletic season, however, athletes in both groups showed an increase of irregular cycles and absence of cycles. Consistent with their early history, the premenarche starters had fewer cycles and a longer time period between cycles (52 days) than the postmenarche starters (35 days). The control group had a normal pattern of regular menstrual cycles throughout the season.

What explained the menstrual differences between the athletes and control subjects and between the athletes who had begun training before and after menarche? One of the reasons could be that the athletes who had irregular or no menstrual cycles were at or below the minimum weight for their height necessary for the maintenance of cycles in nonathletic women; this is what we had found in the ballet dancers. Among the runners, those who trained before menarche were leaner than those who trained after menarche. I used ultrasound measurements of subcutaneous fat thickness of the midthigh, fat over the hip joint, and alongside the umbilicus (belly button) to supplement estimated level of overall fatness based on height and weight. The top-ranking athletes had very little subcutaneous fat at these sites compared to control subjects, who had as much as four or five inches of subcutaneous fat at these sites.

You couldn't always tell how lean an athlete was by looking at her. Lean athletes who were very muscular could appear chunky, and they generally weighed the same as the control subjects. It was only when we measured their fatness levels in later studies with total body water and then directly with MRI that we could confirm the significantly lower fatness of the athletes, even when they weighed the same as nonathletic women.

There is an important distinction between these lean athletes who became amenorrheic during the training season, or were amenorrheic even before the season started, and amenorrheic young women with anorexia nervosa, which is a psychogenic disease. Athletes may restrict calories, but they eat without phobia, and much of the food they eat is high in carbohydrates. Athletes also do not have a distorted body image as do anorectics. An anorectic girl can be so thin her rib cage shows, but when she looks in the mirror she thinks her body is fat. Many athletes, however, do share with anorectics an obsession about being fat, particularly in the thighs and abdomen.

RESUMPTION OF MENSTRUAL CYCLES

The time it takes to resume or start cycles depends on how long a girl or woman has been without cycles and how lean she is. The time can be short: take the swimmer described in chapter 1, who turned her cycles on and off with a five-pound weight change in just a month. I met quite a few gymnasts who told me they turned cycles on and off with just a three-pound weight change in very short time intervals. These athletes were usually at a weight close to their minimum weight for height.

But the time interval can also be long. One of the swimmers, now 20 years old, who hadn't had a cycle for six years, had a different experience. She had had menarche relatively late, at age 14, and then became amenorrheic as she trained on one team or another year-round. She was muscular, looking chunky rather than thin. She pulled a tendon, so she had to stop team training. Like all the athletes, she was very cooperative about the research. When I asked her would she please let me know when her cycles returned and her weight at the time, she said she would be delighted to do so. Then she took a semester off and went to Spain.

She didn't return until more than a year later. "It took ten months to get my cycles back, and I forgot to write down the weight at the time," she told me when we met again. "But I can see you're looking at me, Dr. Frisch," she added. Indeed I was, because she looked too thin and I couldn't believe she had regular cycles. When I asked her about her regularity, she replied, "Oh, I don't have any cycles now. I joined a bicycle team when I came back, and I've been training hard to get in shape."

In general, the length of time to resumption or commencement of normal cycles is related to how long cycles have been stopped, how much the athlete reduces her activity, and whether she has a reasonable diet both for total calories and calories from fat. Athletes who had left the team at the end of the season, which lasted six months, would come to see us, and almost all of them complained of a new little roll of fat below the umbilicus and around the hips. That's where estrogen puts fat.

DIFFERENCES IN FOOD INTAKE IN PRE- AND POSTMENARCHEAL ATHLETES

I was curious about the athletes' diet, and there was very little information on the subject. A subset of thirteen swimmers and eleven runners kept a seven-day food diary for us to analyze. They recorded what and how much they ate and drank every day. The data were then analyzed by computer. We were surprised to find that the eating habits of athletes, both swimmers and runners, who had started their training before menarche differed from those who had started training after menarche. Remember, the diets were being recorded four or five years after menarche for the premenarcheal group, and about six or seven years after menarche for the postmenarcheal group.

We found that the diet of premenarcheal starters had fewer calories, less protein, a lower percentage of calories from fat, less total fat, less saturated fat, and less calcium than that of their postmenarcheal-trained teammates. We're not sure why the premenarcheal athletes differed in what they ate. Maybe it was because they wanted to be thinner; the premenarcheal runners, but not the swimmers, did weigh less than their postmenarcheal teammates. Other researchers have found that long-term, well-trained athletes eat like our early-trained athletes, especially by eating little total fat and saturated fat. Whatever the reason for such eating habits, they're very good for long-term health.

POSITIVE BIOLOGICAL EFFECTS
OF ATHLETIC TRAINING

Moderate, regular exercise at the start of the adolescent growth spurt, when girls are about 9 years old, can delay menarche from age 12.5 to about 15—the average age of menarche about a century ago. Back then children grew more slowly, probably because of lower-fat diets and the incidence of various childhood diseases. Our athletes, in contrast, were healthy and strong; they apparently had just been leaner longer. This pays off in long-term female health, as I will explain.

What is so great about menarche at age 12, anyway? When I asked this question at a symposium, I was surprised to find that it was upsetting to some members of the audience, and I heard some strange, emotional responses. "It's natural," they said. "Well, a century ago, it was natural to have menarche at age 15 in Europe," I replied. "And in 1900 it was natural at age 14 in the United States." When girls grow more slowly on lower-fat diets, and they exercise moderately, it's natural to have a later menarche. The earlier menarche of fatter girls increases both the risk of breast cancer later in life and the risk of a teenage pregnancy too early in life.

There's another advantage of delayed menarche, as we and others found. When a girl has menarche late, about age 15, regular ovulatory cycles do not start as early and as regularly after menarche as they do in a girl who has menarche at about age 12. The early maturers can start regular ovulatory cycles six months after menarche. Late maturers usually do not have regular ovulatory cycles until two or three years after menarche. That brings girls up to ages 17 and 18 before they ovulate at regular intervals, much closer to the age of reason and maturity. Teenage pregnancies at present occur even among girls who are only 12 to 15 years old. Pregnancy at these ages is especially dangerous and unfortunate for both the mother and the infant because the physical growth of the girls is not completed until age 16 to 18. In addition to the psychological immaturity at ages 12 to 15, there is thus the physical immaturity.

OTHER POSITIVE EFFECTS OF ATHLETIC TRAINING

As we collected data on our athletes month after month, we learned something else about them that would be just as important as the physical delay of menarche. Our athletes had great team spirit. They had high self-esteem and took pride in their athletic skill and their place on the team. They also turned to one another and to their coach when they had problems. It occurred to me that this kind of camaraderie would be a great help to adolescent girls, especially if they felt alienated and lacked support from family or friends.

I'd been told that in one high school, teenage pregnancies were frequent among nonathletes but rare among girls on athletic teams. Teenage pregnancy is a problem that pervades all socioeconomic levels and is present in the suburbs as well as in the cities. A broad program to interest young girls and boys in moderate, well-supervised exercise may be a constructive approach to the problem. We learned from physical education teachers and guidance counselors that even the idea of exercise is foreign to the daughters or mothers of some ethnic and cultural groups. "These girls wouldn't set foot in a gym," one counselor said. But they don't have to. Schools could offer jazz dancing, or other kinds of physical activity; exercise doesn't have to involve team sports. But the increase in self-confidence, the pride in physical fitness, the support of the group, and the feeling of belonging to the group are important aspects of whatever physical activities are offered. Psychological support may be a preventive factor.

Athletes at even young ages take great pride in being physically fit: they don't like to gain excessive weight or to become fat. This can translate into long-term benefits to health—being leaner, for example, reduces the risk of cardiovascular disease and diabetes. And as I will describe in detail in the next chapter, athletic training started in high school or earlier is associated with a lower lifetime occurrence of cancer in the breast and reproductive system and of late-onset diabetes, all serious diseases of women in their fifties and older. Athletic activity also increases the density of the bones. Young girls who exercise regularly and moderately during the adolescent years could enter the menopausal period with a greater bone mass.

A 19-YEAR-OLD RUNNER WHO LOOKED ONLY 12

A girl was running around the track when I walked into the Harvard field house with the coach one day. The runner was about four and a half feet tall and couldn't have weighed more than sixty-five pounds. How nice of Harvard to let elementary school children use the track, I thought. "Meet Tracy," said the coach. "She's one of our fastest runners." Tracy (not her real name) was a junior at Harvard. I learned her history when she came to us for her measurements. Tracy had attended a ballet boarding school when she was about 10 years old. Practice sessions at the school usually ended shortly before dinnertime, and Tracy was never hungry then, so she skipped that meal—and many others. Tracy had never had a menstrual cycle, and she had no breasts; she looked like a charming, prepubertal 12-year-old.

I already knew that the adolescent growth spurt can be delayed if a girl stays too thin, and Tracy was a clear example. She was unconcerned, but her parents were very concerned. They wrote, saying that Tracy had been examined by a doctor and he couldn't find anything wrong. "Everyone in our family has a normal height and weight, including Tracy's adult sisters," they wrote. "Could you please have her checked by a doctor in Boston?" After the most careful examination, that doctor couldn't find anything wrong, either. I was fascinated with Tracy's evening temperature records. They never rose above 96°F, and they fluctuated down to 94°F. Her temperature pattern reminded me of the anorexia patients I had studied at Children's Hospital.

After this series of checks, Tracy's doctor at home said she would have to have a CAT scan of her brain unless she ate and gained weight. So Tracy ate. She grew to the normal height and weight of a 19-year-old, and she "developed," as the coach told us sadly. (Tracy wasn't on the team at the time, so I didn't have the chance to measure her.) The coach was sad, I knew, because once Tracy developed a mature body composition, she gained a lot of fat. Alas, she never again ran as fast as she did when she was that lean, prepubertal size. After she graduated, the coach told me, she married and had two healthy children.

Another unusual young woman called me up for help; she was a body builder. She didn't run or jog or dance; she just exercised to "get in shape" for competition. She became very lean, as you can see from figure 12 below, and her menstrual cycles stopped. Measurements of her reproductive hormones showed them to be very low, as would be expected from her excessive leanness. Normal cycles returned when she stopped training and "went out of shape," as she phrased it.

EARLY DIETING AND STUNTED HEIGHT

Researchers of children who diet obsessively during the early years of the adolescent growth spurt, beginning on average at age 9 for girls and age 11 for boys, found that there is a critical time in the growth spurt in height. After that critical time, height does not "catch up" and make up for the lost growth, even if the girls and boys have gained weight into the normal range for their age. These children become stunted in height and do not attain their genetic potential. Parents of young children on teams need to watch out for overzealous coaches

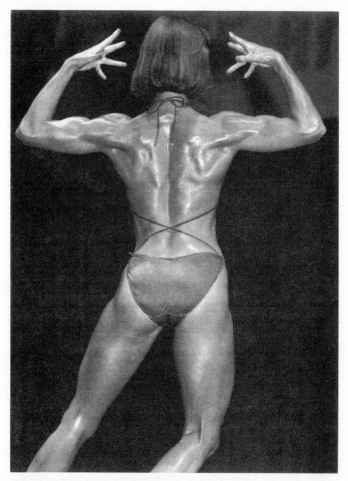

Figure 12. The body builder pictured above stopped menstruating when she was "in shape" for competition. She contacted me to have her hormone levels checked because, as she said, "I don't jog. I don't run. I just build up my muscles." As would be expected from her very lean body composition, her levels of estrogen, follicle-stimulating hormones (FSH), and luteinizing hormone (LH), were low, similar to the levels in amenorrheic athletes who train intensively (those who run more than twenty miles a week, for example). When she went "out of shape," losing muscle and gaining fat, her menstrual cycles were restored.

who care more for winning than for the long-term health of their athletes. Boy wrestlers are particularly at risk because at competition time some coaches urge the boys to lose weight before the weigh-in time that determines whether they are on a lightweight or heavyweight team. If a boy is really a heavyweight but loses a lot of weight so he will seem to be a lightweight, he has an advantage. Sometimes it's not only the coach who encourages such a practice. I met a coach at a sports medicine conference who was very discouraged to find that the parents thought he should urge his adolescent wrestlers to lose weight, even though he told them how bad it was for their health and normal growth. "Anything to win" was the parents' attitude.

Our English Channel Swimmer and the Effect of Protective Fat

One day I was waiting at Logan Airport in Boston for the arrival of a flight from London. I held a large sign with Dr. H. Smith (not his real name) printed on it. A young woman walked in front of me, then turned and with flashing eyes and rising voice asked, "Why are you meeting my husband?" "He's bringing urine and blood samples collected from Sharon Beckman, our English Channel swimmer, after she landed on the rocks of Calais a couple of days ago," was my reply. The lady understandably looked amazed.

Her husband emerged from customs at that moment, carrying a white box with the samples I was waiting for and bringing greetings from our London collaborator, Dr. George Hall, who had accompanied Sharon across the channel in the pilot boat. Dr. Hall was an anesthesiologist interested in body composition. I met him through a friend of his who was working on the development of lean pigs; lean pigs, like a lot of other lean mammals, are very poor reproducers. Many paths converge when you work on the reproductive problems of lean athletes.

When Sharon Beckman, the captain of the Harvard swim team, told me she was planning to swim the English Channel,

I did my best to talk her out of it. But Sharon had made up her mind: she wanted to swim it "because it is there," she said. Since I couldn't talk her out of it, I asked Sharon if I could study the effects of her daily training in Boston Harbor and the effects of the nine-hour swim on her reproductive hormones, on the hormones controlling stress, and on metabolism.

To swim the English Channel, a swimmer sometimes has to gain weight: fat protects against the cold water of the channel. I took Sharon to the Environmental Medicine Center at the U.S. Army Research Institute, where technicians could measure the changes in her core temperature after she swam in water that was as cold as the channel. After the test, she was told to gain about 12 pounds (5.5 kg) to improve heat conservation during the swim; otherwise, she would not last the nine hours in the water. At 154 pounds (70 kg), Sharon was already rather heavy, but she was also tall, 68 inches (173 cm), and muscular, so she did not look plump. Sharon proceeded to eat foods high in carbohydrates and gained weight over a period of about six months while she trained.

As far as I knew, coordinated metabolic and reproductive changes had not been studied over a period of time for a female athlete. My research plan was to assay a whole battery of substances: ketone bodies, glycerol, C-peptide, 3 methyl histidine, thyroid hormones (all of these for metabolic assays); diurnal urinary catecholamines (for stress assessment); and the reproductive hormones and adrenal androgens (for reproductive function) in relation to the stages of training and to the channel swim. The resulting 1984 paper in the medical journal *Metabolism* had nine coauthors because I put together a team from three laboratories at Harvard Medical School to do the study. I kept in shape myself running around to all the labs with samples once the study was under way.

I collected samples of blood and urine during the six-month training period prior to the channel swim in August, immediately after the swim (that's when Dr. Hall climbed on the rocks of Calais and collected the samples that Dr. Smith brought me), and in the postswim untrained, baseline period. Sharon kept a record of her daily temperature and a history of her menstrual cycles over the whole time. Sharon took containers to the law office where she was working so that she could collect urine samples during the day. Never was there a more cooperative and dedicated subject.

At the beginning of training in March, Sharon swam four miles in a pool, about an hour and a half, each day. By June and early July, she swam five to six miles, three and a half to four hours daily. Starting in April, part of her training was in Boston Harbor, where the water temperature was about 50°F (10°C). This was before Boston Harbor was cleaned up; after heavy rains, sewage would overflow into the harbor, as Sharon found out. She would bike down to the Boston Harbor beach from her law office job, get a little towel from the lady in the booth, and then take off into the waters of the harbor, with nobody else around. I worried about her, but she seemed to think it was a very natural thing to do. She had trained for competitive distance swimming since she was 10 years old.

While Sharon was at the U.S. Army Research Center, technicians measured her relative fatness by underwater weighing. Essentially, the density of the body is measured by how much water is displaced, and from the density you can estimate the lean mass and fat. Sports-medicine researchers used this method almost exclusively, whereas medical researchers used measurements of body water. Underwater weighing can be very useful; for example, in World War II, the navy rejected very fit football players because, they said, the men were overweight. By using underwater weighing, the navy learned that the men were not obese; they were very muscular, and muscles weigh more than fat.

A lot of assumptions are made, however, when that method is applied to women. It was very interesting to learn that Sharon's body composition was 20 percent fat by the underwater method but 30 percent fat by equations based on body water or on neutron activation, another indirect method. During the entire time we studied athletes, controversy raged over measurements and estimates of fatness because the measurements were indirect. We also used the direct method of ultrasound to measure the subcutaneous fat of Sharon's abdominal wall at the level of the belly button; in two separate measurements, before the swim it was 11 and 13 millimeters thick. Her subcutaneous fat thickness on the thigh measured 8 millimeters. Our very lean runners had only about 1 to 2 millimeters of subcutaneous fat on the abdomen. I thought the 30 percent number for overall fatness was probably more accurate than the 20 percent estimate.

Postswim Measurements and Cycles

Sharon completed the channel swim of 25 miles (40 km) on August 28, 1982, in nine hours and six minutes. She said one of the biggest problems was avoiding the debris and garbage floating in the English Channel. The assays for the metabolic products we studied showed that fat breakdown was the principal source of energy for the swim, as has been found for prolonged aerobic exercise in men. During the training period there was a fall in insulin secretion and a decline in the urinary catecholamines, which reflect function of the adrenal gland and the sympathetic nervous system; this was also similar to the responses to progressive athletic training in men. After the swim, there was a sharp rise in the substances that are usually observed after severe stress, during surgery or an injury. Nearly normal levels of these stress signals were observed twelve hours after the swim, a remarkably rapid restoration time.

During Sharon's training from March through August, her menstrual cycles of five days' duration continued at 24- to 29-day intervals. The temperature records showed, however, that she had a short luteal phase (a sign of a change in the hormones controlling ovulation) in June and July. In August before the swim, there was no midcycle rise in temperature; the cycle was therefore probably anovulatory. But a normal menstrual flow of five days' duration began the day after the swim. The November postswim, post-training cycle was probably ovulatory. The suppression of ovulation in the cycle immediately before the swim is consistent with other evidence that intense exercise can suppress ovulation.

But with so long a period of intense exercise and so much psychological stress, Sharon might have expected to have no cycles at all, like other very lean swimmers. An explanation may be that Sharon had a high percentage of body fat relative to her lean mass, as was indicated by her ultrasound measurements and her estimated body composition. I couldn't find any other data on menstrual cycles of female channel swimmers, so we can't compare Sharon's experience with the experience of other women who have a craze to swim the channel. (Sharon's results do make one wonder about the sperm count before, during, and after the swim for the many men who swim the channel.) Two months after the cessation of training, Sharon had normal levels of the hormones that control ovulation and a normal ovulatory cycle, demonstrating the reversibility of the effects of the exercise.

Sharon went on to attend the University of Michigan Law School, serve as editor in chief of her school's law review, and clerk for two distinguished jurists, including U.S. Supreme Court Justice Sandra Day O'Connor. Sharon is now an assistant professor at Boston College Law School and still swims regularly. She has two young daughters.

9 Exercise and Lower Risk of Breast Cancer

The Alumnae Health Study

I knew that those super lean, exercising women whose menstrual cycles had stopped could start them again by regaining body fat. But I didn't know whether there were serious effects later in life on the general or reproductive health of girls and women, such as the ballet dancers and athletes I had studied, who had turned off their cycles by being too lean.

Many Questions to Answer

Nobody else seemed to know, either, and there was a long list of unanswered, important questions:

• When menarche is delayed until age 18, 19, or 20, is the woman's fertility affected later?

• If an athlete has irregular cycles or no cycles for a period of months or years, will there be any effects on her long-term general or reproductive health?

• Will a former athlete be more likely to have bone fractures during and after menopause?

• Does regular, moderate exercise in college or earlier affect the risk of sex-hormone-sensitive cancers—breast cancer and cancers of the reproductive system—later in life?

• The incidence of diabetes and non-reproductive-system

cancers is known to rise during and after menopause; is the incidence the same for former athletes and nonathletes?

To find the answers to these and a host of other questions, my collaborators and I studied 5,398 female college graduates: 2,622 were former college athletes and 2,776 were their nonathletic classmates. Because we used alumnae as subjects, we were able to recruit a very large number of women with a wide age range, and we were able to verify past athletic activity for the athletic alumnae. Also, the control subjects for the athletes had to be from a similar age group and background; sedentary classmates as control subjects for each age bracket provided the solution. College alumnae offices, moreover, keep excellent, up-to-date records of their graduates. (Only 3.5 percent of our questionnaires were nondeliverable.)

Male college athletes had already been studied in comparison to nonathletes, and the athletic men had superior health later in life. As far as I knew, ours was the first study comparing female college athletes and nonathletes. Would the happy outcome for the men be true for the women?

We studied graduates of eight colleges and two universities: Barnard, Bryn Mawr, Mount Holyoke, Radcliffe, Smith, Springfield, Vassar, Wellesley, the University of Southern California, and the University of Wisconsin. All the institutions gave us permission to contact the alumnae through their athletic departments and alumnae offices.

COLLECTING FAMILY AND MEDICAL HISTORIES

What did we ask? Fourteen pages of questions—with lots of space for the answers. It wasn't one of those "yes or no" questionnaires; we wanted detailed life histories.

We asked about medical history, reproductive history, exercise history, diet, menarche, menopause, and family history. We included many questions about each woman's height, weight, weight changes over the years, current diet, smoking history, births, pregnancy outcomes, problems with infertility, contraceptive use, medications, hospitalizations, other medical history, family history of cancer and diabetes—

everything we could think of that would help us analyze the health status of the former athletes compared to that of the nonathletes. Our respondents, with very few exceptions, answered all the questions.

Collaborators on the project included physicians from Harvard Medical School's Department of Medicine and Department of Obstetrics and Gynecology, a nutritionist, and experts in athletics. We wanted to be sure we were asking the most important lifetime health questions. Dr. Grace Wyshak was the biostatistician of the project.

In 1982 we mailed the questionnaire to 7,559 alumnae—half were former college athletes as verified by their college, and half were sedentary classmates. Skeptics said that not many women would take the time to answer so many detailed, open-ended questions. Also, they predicted that alumnae might be offended by questions on the use of contraceptives, infertility, or menopausal history and refuse to answer.

The skeptics were wrong. We had a remarkable response: 5,398 women, or 71.4 percent of the alumnae, ranging in age from 20 to 80, filled out and returned the questionnaire. Of the 5,398 respondents, 2,622 (48.6 percent) were athletes in college and 2,776 (51.4 percent) were nonathletes. Some respondents even called to offer more information. I remember one call in particular: my office phone rang, and a voice on the other end of the line said, "Thanks for the questionnaire—and let me tell you more. No one ever cared about my medical problems before." She did tell me a lot more! Replies came from as far away as Beijing, China (with an apology for the delayed response—the questionnaire had been forwarded from Kansas City).

Our cover letter to the alumnae did not state that we would be comparing athletes and nonathletes, as that would have biased the study. We said that we were interested in the long-term health of female college graduates. All the data were kept confidential, and no name was ever used in any of the results. A code number was given to each questionnaire upon receipt, and the questionnaire was separated from the name during the analysis of the data.

We made one exception to our rule against breaking the code. We received a questionnaire that had *HELP* written in block letters down the side of the page containing the questions on medical problems. In that instance, we broke the code to find out who was so desperate. The respondent, we learned, had a serious unsolved medical problem and lived in a small town far from a hospital or medical center. We consulted a specialist about her problem, then sent her the name and address of the facility closest to her where she could get help. Otherwise, our analysis was completely anonymous.

Former College Athletes: Moderate Exercisers

The former college athletes we studied were moderate exercisers, not marathoners or Olympic-level athletes. A woman qualified as an athlete if she had been on a varsity, house, or intramural team for at least one year. For the alumnae in their seventies and eighties there were no female athletic teams in college, so we categorized them by a more flexible standard (for example, a distinction such as the award of a college letter was acceptable evidence of being an athlete).

Team sports had to be what our physician athletic advisor (and former Olympic gold medal skater) Dr. Tenley Albright called "energy intensive": for example, basketball, crew, field hockey, soccer, squash, swimming, tennis, track, or volleyball. Dance, fencing, softball, and gymnastics were also included. Team training had to be regular, at least two practice sessions a week during the academic year. Some of the younger alumnae ran or jogged; they were categorized as athletes if they ran at least two miles a day, five days a week, regularly. About 67 percent of our former college athletes were on more than one college team, and more than 80 percent were on a team two or more years. About 40 percent played on a team all four years.

I had learned from our earlier studies of athletes that it was important to find out when in their lives the athletes had begun regular exercise, especially whether they had begun before or after menarche. So we asked the alumnae how old they had been when they began athletic training, and we requested all the details about it: the type of training, whether it was year-round or seasonal, and whether it was more or less rigorous than their college training. We found that of the former college athletes, 82 percent had also participated on an athletic team in high school or earlier, compared to 25 percent of their nonathletic classmates.

We also asked for details about current exercise and found that 75 percent of the former athletes were still exercising regularly. Interestingly, 57 percent of the nonathletic alumnae reported they were now exercising regularly as well. These alumnae were intelligent women, and they must have heeded the advice of numerous magazine and newspaper articles emphasizing the importance of exercise for good health.

ATHLETIC EXERCISE AND LOWER RISK OF BREAST AND REPRODUCTIVE-SYSTEM CANCERS

It took almost two years to analyze our detailed data, but when we were finished, we had a very exciting result: we discovered that women who had participated in organized athletic activity in college had a significantly lower lifetime occurrence (prevalence) rate of breast cancer and reproductive-system cancers than their sedentary classmates did (see figure 13 below). These cancers account for more than 40 percent of all cancers in women. As we reported in the *British Journal of Cancer* in 1985, the lifetime occurrence rate of breast cancer in nonathletes was almost twice that of the athletes. We also found that the lifetime occurrence rate of breast cancer in nonathletes showed a sharp rise during the perimenopausal period (around ages 49 and 50), like women in other Western, well-nourished populations, whereas athletes had a less steep rise in this period.

Following standard procedure when many factors are involved, our statistical analysis took into account the significant risk factors for breast cancer such as age, history of cancer in the family, and age of menarche. When we looked at family history, we learned that breast cancer in the mother

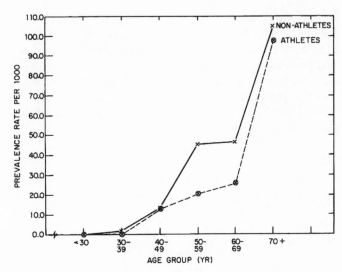

Figure 13. Prevalence (lifetime occurrence rate) of breast cancer for athletes and nonathletes by age group. From R. E. Frisch et al., "Lower Prevalence of Breast Cancer and Cancers of the Reproductive System among Former College Athletes Compared to Nonathletes," *British Journal of Cancer* 52 (1985): 885. Reprinted with permission of the publisher Churchill Livingstone.

was similar for the two groups, 6.9 percent in the athletes and 7.5 percent in the nonathletes. Breast cancer in a sister was 1.2 percent in both groups.

Former college athletes in every age group also had lower prevalence rates of cancers of the uterus, ovary, cervix, and vagina compared to the nonathletes (see figure 14 below). For nonathletes, the prevalence rate of cancers of the reproductive system was about two and a half times that of college athletes. Notice in figure 14 the steep rise in the prevalence rate of reproductive-system cancers in the menopausal years among the nonathletes compared to the athletes.

Dr. Wyshak and our team also published the finding that former college athletes had a significantly lower lifetime oc-

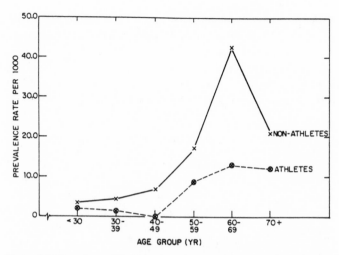

Figure 14. Prevalence (lifetime occurrence rate) of reproductive-system cancers for athletes and nonathletes by age group. From R. E. Frisch et al., "Lower Prevalence of Breast Cancer and Cancers of the Reproductive System among Former College Athletes Compared to Nonathletes," *British Journal of Cancer* 52 (1985): 887. Reprinted with permission of the publisher Churchill Livingstone.

currence of *benign* tumors of the breast and reproductive system.

As with the breast cancer data analysis, the comparison of the rates between the former athletes and nonathletes took into account the many factors that can affect the risk of reproductive-system cancers, including age, family history of cancer, age of menarche, number of pregnancies, use of estrogen in the menopausal period, and smoking. (We had detailed information on all these factors from our fourteen-page questionnaire.) The family history of cancer for all female blood relatives did not differ much between the two groups, but we were surprised at the high percentages: 49.8 for former athletes and 51.7 for the nonathletes. The percentages of cancer in the mother were similar: 18.1 for former athletes and 17.9 for nonathletes.

As far as we knew, ours was the first study to report the relationship of physical activity to the risk of sex-hormone-sensitive cancers in women. Our results were reported nationwide by the press. I was interviewed by Cable News Network and various television stations and was delighted to discuss results so important to women's long-term health.

IT'S NOT TOO LATE TO START EXERCISING

Suppose you didn't start exercising when you were young or even in college. Should you start now? Women who had heard about our research called and asked this very question. "I'm twenty years old; is it too late for me to do anything about exercise?" I could not give a definitive answer at the time because our research did not specifically cover that question. We did not know whether young women who began regular exercise in, say, their early twenties or thirties and kept it up regularly until they entered the perimenopausal and menopausal period would have a lower risk of breast cancer and reproductive-system cancers. But, I told them, the average age of menopause—52, with a standard deviation (variation around the average) of plus or minus 5 years—was old enough to allow for a nice, long time to do regular exercise and stay relatively lean. They had nothing to lose (except excess fat, perhaps)—and a lot to gain—by exercising. "Who knows?" I would add. "Maybe twenty or thirty years of regular exercise will reduce the risk of breast cancer and reproductive-system cancers in the menopausal years."

Now it is well known that being lean later in life reduces the risk of heart attack, stroke, and late-onset diabetes. And because exercise increases bone density, women who exercise regularly enter menopause with a larger bone mass, which reduces their risk of bone fracture. Regular exercise has so many advantages that it is a lifestyle to adopt at any age. Moreover, according to a recent study by Leslie Bernstein and her collaborators at the University of Southern California, women age 40 and younger who spend just one to three hours a week exercising reduce their risk of breast cancer by about 30 percent compared to inactive women. A steady level of physical activity of four or more hours a week reduces the breast cancer risk by about 50 percent. The moral of the story? Find a physical activity you enjoy and do it regularly.

WHY EXERCISE LOWERS THE RISK OF THESE CANCERS

Why did the former athletes have a lower lifetime occurrence of breast cancer and reproductive-system cancers? At present we can only speculate about the reasons. Cancer develops over a long period of time, commonly twenty years or more. Many factors can affect the initiation and growth of a cancer.

At the time of the study, we could rule out some reasons for lower incidence of these cancers among the former athletes. Genetic factors were unlikely, as the former athletes and nonathletes had similar family histories of cancer. Also, we had strong evidence against selection or reporting biases, because the prevalence rates of breast cancer and reproductive-system cancers for the nonathletic alumnae accorded with the data for the general population.

We could also rule out a difference in fertility, as former athletes and nonathletes had similar lifetime fertility data. The athletes had 2.2 live births on average, the nonathletes 2.1 live births, and the average age of the mother at first birth was 27 in both groups. The two groups also had similar pregnancy histories: the athletes did not have more pregnancy losses. The percentages of women who had ever had a pregnancy were almost identical, 61.9 for athletes and 61.1 percent for nonathletes, as were the number of pregnancies (2.8 and 2.7, respectively). These numbers of pregnancies and live births are typical of middle-class and upper-class women in the general population. The data answered another question: whether fertility later in life was affected by a delay in menarche or by earlier episodes of amenorrhea or irregular menstrual cycles. Apparently, later fertility was unaffected; in fact, one former athlete who had menarche at age 28 went on to bear seven children.

One factor that does help to explain the difference in cancer risk has to do with the effects of relative fatness. Both early menarche and late menopause are related to greater relative fatness, and previous research by others has shown that a higher risk of cancer of the breast and of the endometrium are associated with early menarche, late menopause, and greater relative fatness. Comparing the relative fatness of the former athletes and nonathletes, we found that former athletes were leaner at every age than the nonathletes. Then, as would be expected if they were leaner, the former athletes had menarche later and menopause earlier than did the nonathletes, whose ages matched those of the general population. The former athletes had menarche at age 13.0 on average, while the nonathletes had menarche at age 12.7. The former athletes had menopause at age 51.3 on average, and the nonathletes had menopause at age 52.0. Although these differences are not large, they are statistically significant.

A related explanation is that the small but significant difference in relative leanness between athletes and nonathletes, which we found in every age group from 20 to 80, may have existed long term, before the college years. It may also have been larger at earlier ages since more than 80 percent of the former athletes were members of teams in secondary school or earlier compared to only 24 percent of their nonathletic classmates. Early maturers who are fatter than late maturers have higher concentrations of estrogen in their blood than do leaner, later-maturing girls both at menarche and *after* menarche. I learned this important fact from Dr. Dan Apter of Helsinki, Finland, at a recent conference on exercise and the risk of breast cancer.

In general, fatness and leanness may have a lot to do with our cancer-risk results. Fatness is associated with an increased conversion of androgens (male hormones) to estrogens (female hormones). Fatness also is associated with the metabolism of estrogen to more potent forms, which in turn is associated with an increased risk of breast cancer. The more potent forms of estrogen may result in more cell division in reproductive tissues. Whenever there is cell division, there is a chance of a mistake in the duplication of genes, and such mistakes may increase the risk that a cell will become cancerous. Leanness, in contrast, is associated with an increased level of nonpotent estrogen, which is relatively inactive. It is as if the reproductive system is put on "idle." Cells of the reproductive system do not increase at the normal rapid rate.

MEASURING BODY FAT DIRECTLY WITH MRI

Some researchers argued that the degree of fatness might not affect the metabolism of estrogen to a potent or nonpotent form. My collaborators and I had the good fortune to be able to measure body fat directly in *living* athletes and nonathletes and also to measure how much of the nonpotent estrogen was present in their blood.

We collaborated with Dr. Bruce Rosen of Massachusetts General Hospital to measure body fat directly with MRI. By computer you can count the pixels (units of measurement) of fat in the image of a particular area; in the MRI picture below (fig. 15), the bright white areas are body fat. This was the first time MRI was used to compare the amount of fat directly under the skin (subcutaneous fat) and inside the body cavity (visceral fat) in athletic and nonathletic women. We measured subcutaneous and visceral fat at six regional body sites; they are indicated by the dots and lines on the *Aphrodite of Kyrene* figure, also shown below (fig. 16). Numbers refer to vertebrae in the spinal column.

What the MRI pictures told us was that the athletic young women had one-third less fat than their sedentary classmates although the body weights of the two groups were similar. (Remember, muscle is heavier than fat, and the athletes had a lot of muscle.) At each of the six regional sites, athletes had significantly less fat than the control subjects; you can see this in the MRI pictures of one site, the thigh of an Olympic rower compared to that of a control subject. Note the larger size of muscle in the rower's thigh, as well as the decrease in fat. The athletes wept when they saw they still had that much fat!

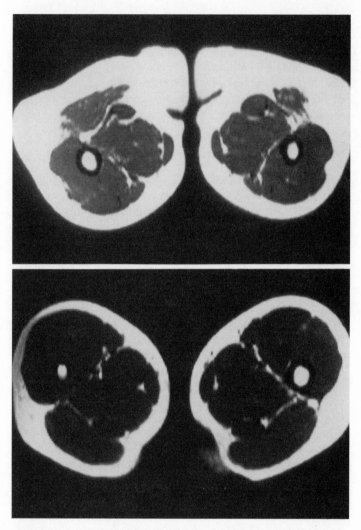

Figure 15. MRI cross-sectional scans of the midthigh of a 20-year-old nonathlete (above) and of a 22-year-old Olympic rower (below) during intensive training. Note the athlete's large amount of muscle and small amount of fat compared to the nonathlete.

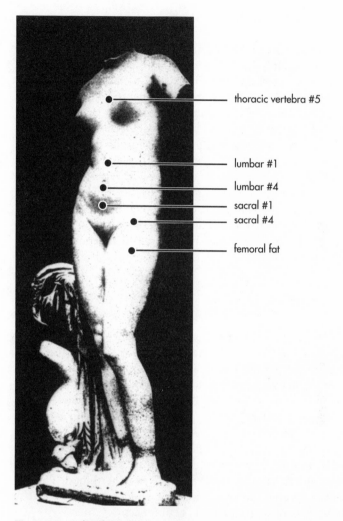

thoracic vertebra #5

lumbar #1

lumbar #4

sacral #1

sacral #4

femoral fat

Figure 16. *Aphrodite of Kyrene*, showing location of MRI measurements of subcutaneous and visceral fat at six regional body sites. Numbers refer to vertebrae in the spinal column. Athletes in our study lost body fat at all sites shown above; the amount of fat they lost differed from nonathletes depending on the site. The picture of the statue comes from Kenneth Clark's art book, *The Nude*; no medical texts I consulted had a suitable figure. Copyright 1956 by the Trustees of the National Gallery of Art. Reprinted by permission of Princeton University Press.

An unexpected finding about differences in the amount of fat lost among the six regional sites also dismayed the athletes: the largest difference between athletes and control subjects was in the regions with the least fat per unit volume, the region of the breast (thoracic vertebra 5 in the figure above) and above the umbilicus (lumbar 1), not the sites where the athletes wanted less fat, around the abdomen (lumbar 4, sacral 1, and sacral 4) and in the thigh (femoral fat). Interestingly, in premenopausal women, thigh fat reportedly has a reduced response to insulin and to catecholamines (hormones secreted by the adrenal medulla), both of which control release of energy from fat cells. During pregnancy and lactation this tendency is reversed—that is, fat is made more available for use as energy.[1]

CONFIRMING THE LINK BETWEEN LEANNESS AND NONPOTENT ESTROGEN

Knowing the amount of body fat in each young woman, my doctoral student Rachel Snow (now a researcher at the Medical School of the University of Heidelberg) measured the nonpotent estrogen in each woman and related it to her body fat as quantified by the MRI. The research was done in the laboratory of Dr. Robert Barbieri of Brigham and Women's Hospital in Boston. In 1993 my collaborators and I reported our findings in the *Journal of Clinical Endocrinology and Metabolism:* the greater the leanness of an athlete, the larger the amount of the nonpotent estrogen in her blood. This result supported the hypothesis that leanness contributed to a lower risk of reproductive-system cancers.

Another possible explanation for the former athletes' lower prevalence rates for sex-hormone-sensitive cancers may be that girls who begin to exercise early in life apparently eat differently from other girls. We found that the runners and

1. M. Rebuffé-Scrive, L. Enk, N. Crona, P. Lönnroth, L. Abrahamsson, U. Smith, and P. Björntorp, "Fat Cell Metabolism in Different Regions in Women: Effect of Menstrual Cycle, Pregnancy and Lactation," *Journal of Clinical Investigation* 75 (1985): 1973–76.

swimmers who began their training before menarche ate less fat and less saturated fat later, when they were 19 or 20 years old, than their teammates who had begun their training after menarche. Other researchers have also noted that well-trained athletes, both women and men, eat less fat and less saturated fat. Many are vegetarians or semi-vegetarians. From what we observed, we don't think athletes eat less fat because they figure out that such a diet has lower calories or is more healthful. Their dietary choices seem to be an almost involuntary response to a lifestyle of regular exercise. Whatever the reason, the low-fat diet is a healthful addition to their lifestyle. Although some people still regard the effect of a low-fat diet as controversial, much evidence supports the correlation of a high-fat diet and high intake of saturated fats with an increased risk of breast cancer.

One other fact noted earlier is pertinent to the lower risk observed among the leaner athletes. In fatter women, more of the circulating estrogen is in a free state. This is because the protein that binds estrogen, called sex-hormone-binding globulin, somehow has a diminished capacity to bind to estrogen in fatter women. Hence, there is more unbound, free estrogen, which promotes division of cells of the reproductive system and may increase the risk that a cell will become cancerous.

Adding it all up, we concluded that long-term athletic training establishes a lifestyle that lowers the risk of breast cancer and reproductive-system cancers. Exercise young, benefit young—and benefit later.

Does Exercise Lower Risk of Other Types of Cancer?

After we learned that exercise lowers the risk of sex-hormone-sensitive cancers, we wondered if the former athletes differed from the nonathletes in the lifetime occurrence of non-reproductive-system cancers—those of the digestive system, thyroid gland, bladder, lung, and other sites, and cancers of the blood (including leukemia) and skin (including melanoma).

We divided the cancers into two groups. Class 1 included all cancers except those of the skin, which constituted class 2. We had to group the different types of cancers included in class 1 together because the number of each of these types was not large enough to make comparisons between athletes and nonathletes.

The college athletes had a significantly lower prevalence rate of class 1 cancers than their nonathletic classmates. The risk of developing one of these cancers was three times greater for the nonathletes than for the athletes. Of particular interest was the absence of digestive-system cancers among the former athletes compared to the nonathletes. Other studies have shown a lower risk of colon cancer among men and women who have occupations requiring physical activity. In one of these studies, women in occupations requiring physical activity also had a lower mortality rate from breast cancer than did women whose occupations did not require much physical activity.

We can only speculate about why the athletes had a lower risk of developing class 1 cancers. One possible explanation may be that intense exercise has been reported to stimulate natural immunity by increasing activation of cells of the immune system that can destroy tumor cells.

In contrast to the class 1 cancers, the prevalence rates of the class 2 cancers did not differ significantly between the former athletes and nonathletes. Exposure to sunlight is a major factor for malignant melanoma and other skin cancers, and both groups may have had the same level of exposure to the sun. We do not have an explanation of this result as yet.

Athletic Exercise and Lower Rate of Late-Onset Diabetes

We also wanted to know about the risk of getting diabetes after age 20 because it is one of the serious diseases of women in later life, particularly after menopause. We only wanted to know about cases occurring at or after age 20; then we could see the effects, if any, of the athletic training in college and earlier.

It was already well known that well-trained athletes are more sensitive to insulin. That means the beta cells of the pancreas, which make insulin, don't have to work so hard. Less insulin is needed to store glucose (carbohydrate) as fat and to release fat from fat cells when energy is needed for muscular activity or any of the other life functions of the body. Exercise is often recommended when a patient already has diabetes because it will reduce the amount of insulin needed for the normal functioning of the body.

Checking the family history of diabetes in both groups, we found they were similar: 12 percent for the athletes and 13.5 percent for the nonathletes. But, comparing the prevalence rates for the age groups starting at or after age 20, we found that the former athletes consistently had a lower lifetime occurrence of diabetes than the nonathletes in every age group (except for two cases of diabetes under age 30). The prevalence rate of late-onset diabetes in athletes was 58 percent lower than in nonathletes. Also, the prevalence rate did not increase in athletes until after age 50, ten years later than in the nonathletes (see figure 17 below).

Among the alumnae reporting diabetes occurring at or after age 20, 71 percent reported a family history of diabetes. Note the difference in rate between *all the alumnae* reporting a family history of diabetes (12 percent) and those alumnae who *have diabetes* reporting a family history of diabetes (71 percent). Diabetic nonathletes and diabetic former athletes both had a high percentage reporting a family history of diabetes. Clearly, family history of diabetes is a very important factor in developing the disease.

We checked how many of the diabetic women were obese because obesity, defined as weight greater than 120 percent of ideal body weight, is known to increase the risk of diabetes. None of the diabetic former athletes was obese, but 12.5 percent of the diabetic nonathletes were. The former athletes, even if diabetic, did better on long-term body weight maintenance than did the nonathletes.

Although there has been a lot of research showing that physical exercise helps control already-acquired diabetes,

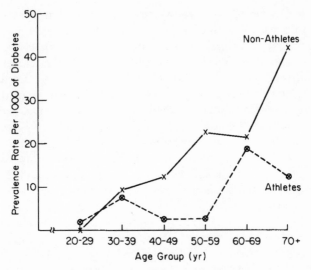

Figure 17. Age-specific prevalence rates (lifetime occurrence rate) per 1,000 women of diabetes among former college athletes and nonathletes. Cases of diabetes occurring before age 20 are not included. From R. E. Frisch et al., "Lower Prevalence of Diabetes in Female Former College Athletes Compared with Nonathletes," *Diabetes* 35 (1986): 1101–1105.

ours was the first study to show that long-term moderate exercise for young girls and *women* reduces the lifetime occurrence after age 20 of non-insulin-dependent diabetes. The most likely reason is that leanness and physical exercise increases the body's sensitivity to insulin. Chalk up another reason to start regular, moderate exercise early in life and keep it up.

No Increase in Bone Fractures — with One Exception

Because intensive exercise can disrupt the menstrual cycle and delay menarche, many people assumed the former athletes would have more bone fractures in the menopausal period. The disruption in menstruation could mean lower estrogen levels over long periods of time, and lower estrogen levels could mean lower bone mass, thereby increasing the risk of osteoporosis (fragile bone due to loss of bone mass). Some researchers found, however, that regular exercise increases bone density. Which effect would be greater in our athletes? Or would the effects cancel each other out? To find out, we studied the lifetime occurrence of bone fractures in our alumnae.

What we found was that the rate of first bone fractures occurring after age 40 (the menopausal and postmenopausal period) did not differ significantly among former college athletes and nonathletes. In fact, fracture rates occurring after age 40 were slightly lower among the former athletes compared to the nonathletes.

When we compared alumnae age 60 and older who had never had a fracture up to age 40, again we found no significant difference in bone fracture rate; the rate for the athletes was 23 percent, the rate for the nonathletes, 26 percent. Starting at age 60, both groups showed a sharp rise in fracture rates of the wrist and hip, fractures that are typical of the menopausal period. The athletes did not have any more fractures than the nonathletes did. The rates for spinal and vertebrae fractures were low in both groups, but showed a rise among those age 70 and older. Young ballet dancers, who also restrict their diet, are reported to have a high rate of spinal and vertebral fractures. Their excessive thinness may increase their risk of such fractures.

All in all, long-term moderate exercise did not result in more bone fractures for the former athletes. Apparently, the increased bone density from exercise compensated for any lower levels of estrogen.

THE COLA–BONE FRACTURE CONNECTION

Having said that, I must immediately point out an exception. A new and unusual finding floated up out of the answers to a question we almost forgot we had asked. Our nutritionist,

Jelia Witschi of the Harvard School of Public Health, had included this question: "Do you drink nonalcoholic carbonated beverages?" She also had asked about alcoholic beverages (wine, beer, hard liquor), coffee, tea, and decaffeinated coffee. In addition, she asked respondents to specify any dietary restrictions: low milk, low fat, low meat, low salt, low calorie, vegetarian, or other.

We asked Dr. Witschi later why she had asked about the nonalcoholic carbonated beverages. Out of curiosity perhaps, she said, because people were drinking so much of the stuff. Or maybe, she thought, she was just being precise in including all kinds of drinks. She couldn't remember exactly, but she wasn't looking for anything special.

We were very surprised to find that the former college athletes in each age group who currently drank nonalcoholic carbonated beverages were at higher risk of experiencing one or more bone fractures during their lifetime compared to former athletes who did not drink these beverages. The difference was highly significant statistically: only one chance in ten thousand that the result was due to chance. It made no difference whether the carbonated beverages were diet drinks (without sugar) or not.

There was even a dose-response relationship between the number of bone fractures at all body sites and the amount of carbonated drinks the athletes consumed. The more they drank, the more bone fractures they had. Only the former athletes showed this effect; the nonathletes could quaff the same stuff and were unaffected.

Of course, Dr. Wyshak, our biostatistician and the person who initially noticed the connection, went looking for a reason. No one had ever observed this link before, as far as we knew. We also were fortunate to be able to consult Dr. Edward Brown of Brigham and Women's Hospital, an expert on bone disease. Dr. Wyshak found that cola drinks contain phosphoric acid, which can leach calcium out of the bones. Bone resorption and bone loss are associated with high phosphorus diets. Some clinicians have reported an increase of bone fractures from occupational exposure to phosphorus, particularly phosphoric acid.

Our results confirmed the adverse effects of a low-milk diet on bone fractures, particularly in the menopausal and postmenopausal athletes. That made sense, because a low-calcium and high-phosphorus intake affect bone loss.

Note that we didn't know what kind of carbonated beverages the alumnae drank. We didn't ask because it never occurred to us that it would matter. We did, however, ask how much they drank; the answer was "a lot." Alumnae who drank nonalcoholic bubbly drinks consumed about fifty gallons a year. That's more than the national average of forty gallons a year. Until we could do a detailed new study, we could only speculate about why the former athletes had more fractures than their sedentary counterparts.

We needed to know exactly what kind of bubbly drinks, and how much, active and inactive girls and boys drank in relation to the number and kind of bone fractures they experienced. We set up a new study to ask those questions of 76 adolescent girls and 51 boys age 8 to 16. We asked exactly what they ate and how much they drank of all kinds of drinks so that we could determine a calcium–phosphorus ratio for each subject. We needed to know how physically active the subjects were, so we asked them to describe their physical activity and rate it on a scale of one (inactive) to five (very vigorous—at least four hour-long sessions a week). A medical questionnaire requested complete data on the occurrence of any bone fractures.

Published in 1993, the results on adolescent boys and girls confirmed our earlier findings on the alumnae, who had ranged in age from 20 to 80. Bone fractures and carbonated beverage consumption were related in adolescent girls. Most of the girls were engaged in moderate to vigorous physical activity. Boys were unaffected.

This time we knew what kinds of carbonated beverages everyone drank, and our findings confirmed the hypothetical connection between cola drinks and increased risk of bone fracture. The results made the national television news, too. Cola drinks, all carbonated beverages combined (including the cola drinks), and low dietary calcium intake were all risk factors for bone fractures. Noncola drinks, other caffeinated drinks, and low-calorie drinks did not affect the risk of bone fracture.

We think the reason that physically active girls are affected by the cola drinks may be that these girls have lower estrogen levels and more nonpotent estrogen because of their leanness than nonactive girls. Consistent with this possibility is that the former college athletes in our earlier studies had a lower lifetime occurrence of breast cancer and reproductive-system cancers compared to the nonathletes. Also, athletic girls drink a lot of diet cola drinks in pursuit of slimness, and the alumnae study indicated that they drank more such drinks than the nonathletic women. (There are too few data on the boys for any explanation.)

Researchers have found that adolescence is a critical time period for bone mass formation. How much bone mass you have is a key determinant of whether you will develop osteoporosis later in life. Our studies indicate that active girls and women should avoid a high consumption of cola drinks in the adolescent years and beyond to lower the risk of osteoporosis in later life. Maybe all women should avoid cola drinks, to be on the safe side.

After we had published an early abstract on the cola–bone fracture connection, we were contacted by the Coca-Cola Company in Atlanta. Could they come up and see us? We said we would be delighted and promptly invited Dr. Edward Brown, the bone expert we had consulted. We all sat around the table in the conference room at Harvard's Population Center and asked questions of one another. One question we researchers wanted to know was how much phosphoric acid was in one can of Coca-Cola. We never got the answer. At the end of the session we asked, wide-eyed, "Doesn't the Coca-Cola Company want to fund more of our research?" No, it didn't.

I had heard of the cola–bone fracture connection even before we published our findings on active young girls. At a sports medicine conference I attended in North Carolina a year or two earlier, an orthopedic surgeon told us of a 25-year-old captain of a university tennis team who was called "Miss Tab" because she drank eight to ten cans of the drink daily. When her bone mass was measured, her tennis arm was normal for a 25-year-old woman (it should have been a greater mass from the exercise), and her other arm had the bone mass of a 70-year-old woman. The speaker recommended that children drink milk. The medical world is so small that years later I learned from Dr. Lawrence Vincent, my collaborator on the ballet-dancer study, that he was the radiologist who had determined Miss Tab's bone mass.

When we published seventeen papers on the alumnae survey results, we sent the titles and references to all the alumnae who had participated in the project. We still receive some letters and phone calls asking whether there have been any new findings. We are grateful to have had the alumnae's careful responses to all the questions, and they were clearly grateful that we had inquired.

FOLLOWING UP ON THE RISK OF BREAST CANCER AMONG ALUMNAE

We recently sent out a fifteen-year follow-up questionnaire to our 5,398 original alumnae subjects who were ages 21 to 80 at time of the original study. Many new factors affecting the long-term health of women have been discovered in the past decade, so there were many new questions on the follow-up questionnaire.

As before, we had an excellent response rate. Of the 4,650 alumnae still living who received the questionnaires, 3,940, or 84.7 percent, responded; former college athletes and nonathletes had similar rates of response. Our results, published in 2000 in the *British Journal of Cancer,* confirmed our earlier findings: former college athletes had a significantly lower risk of breast cancer than the nonathletes. The fifteen-year incidence rate of the former athletes at all ages was 42 percent lower than that of the nonathletes. (The incidence rate is the number of new cases of breast cancer diagnosed in the past fifteen years of athletes and nonathletes per 1,000 women.)

10 Leptin

A New Hormone Made
by Body Fat

The discovery of a new hormone is always news in the scientific world, but leptin made headlines in the front page of the daily news as well. Its discovery in 1994 excited not only scientists but millions of Americans who worry about their excess body fat. They worry with reason, since they are told constantly that being overweight is bad for their health. Too much body fat is associated with serious diseases, including diabetes and cardiovascular disease. Americans spend more than thirty billion dollars a year trying to get thinner. They may succeed for a while, but most gain the excess weight back again in one to five years. Now there is hope on the horizon.

Leptin (from *leptos*, the Greek word for "thin") is a protein hormone made by fat cells; that in itself is something new. How much leptin you have in your blood is closely correlated with how much body fat you have. I was glad for overweight people that leptin might help them achieve a normal weight, but that wasn't why I was excited about leptin. What made me euphoric was that soon after its discovery, leptin was linked to sexual maturation in humans as well as in mice. It was a biochemical link between body fat and reproduction, just the connection I was looking for.

Leptin does two things: it turns down appetite and turns up the rate of energy use. It was discovered by Dr. Jeffrey

Friedman and his colleagues at Rockefeller University in New York when they cloned a mutant *obese* gene in mice. The normal *ob* gene encodes the protein hormone leptin. Mutant *ob/ob* mice lack the normal gene and thus lack leptin; they get fatter and fatter because they keep eating without a stop. When they finally do stop eating, they just lie around rather than running around and working off the fat. Dr. Friedman and his collaborators found that injecting leptin into an over-fat mouse causes the mouse to lose weight and keep it off; the mouse, full of leptin, eats less and runs around more. (Incidentally, the overly fat *ob/ob* mouse is usually infertile.)

Humans, fortunately, also have the fat-controlling gene that encodes leptin. Will leptin do the same for humans? It looks hopeful because leptin slimmed down mice that were fatter just because they were older, and not only because they lacked the normal gene. Women and men also get fatter as they get older beginning at about ages 35 to 40. Look again at figure 7 in chapter 6, and you'll see that the percentage of fat rises in women and men as they age. Even if you eat the same amount of the same foods and your activity level stays the same, more of your weight is fat and less is muscle. That's because your heat production (your metabolic rate) falls as you age, so you burn up less energy. That means you burn fewer calories and store more fat.

Although humans have the fat-controlling gene that encodes leptin, how it works in obese humans is apparently more complicated than in mice. If obese people were like obese mice, they also would have too little leptin. But unexpectedly, it turned out that obese women and men have *too much* leptin in their blood. Apparently, obese humans have something wrong with the receptor for leptin, the molecule leptin is supposed to latch onto. Leptin, like other hormones, works by connecting onto a molecule called the receptor. Receptors carry the hormone with its action message into the brain cell nucleus. Once inside the cell nucleus, that message can start a cascade of biochemical events, or activate other genes involved in the control of the process, or both.

For example, when a mouse has the normal gene for controlling body fat, an increase in body fat causes an increase in leptin. The receptors for leptin then carry the leptin into the nucleus of brain cells, starting the chain of reactions that result in the mouse quitting eating and running around more. Receptors for leptin are found in the hypothalamus, the part of the brain which controls food intake, body temperature, physical activity, emotions—and reproductive ability. The hypothalamus controls all these basic life functions in all mammals from mice to humans. If obese people have a defect in their receptors for leptin or problems with the signaling system, their brain cells would be insensitive to leptin's regulatory function.

Leptin, the Regulator of Body Fat

Though problems remain to be solved in humans with the signaling system for the gene that encodes leptin, the gene has exciting implications. It tells us, for example, that the brain has a way of keeping track of how much fat the body has so that the brain can regulate body weight. Leptin is now regarded as one of the protein hormones that keep body weight in the normal range over long periods. One way to think of it is that your brain has a "lipostat" that regulates body fat the way a thermostat with a set point for a temperature regulates fluctuations in heat. Leptin is the indicator for the lipostat: it turns on with too much fat and turns off with too little fat. Some people may be obese because their lipostat is "set" too high.

The lipostat I wrote about in chapter 3 was a hypothesis published more than thirty years ago by the great English researcher Gordon C. Kennedy of Cambridge University. Kennedy found that food intake was the signal of puberty (the first estrus) in the rat. He measured the quantity of food a female rat ate in relation to its body weight as it grew up to sexual maturation. Kennedy proposed that how much a female rat ate as it matured was controlled by the amount of fat it stored. His results indicated that a particular level of stored fat could be a signal to the brain that enough energy was stored for successful reproduction, initiating the first estrus in the rat (ovulation and the ability to reproduce). Kennedy thought the message to the brain might be a metabolic, heat-production signal reflecting the amount of body fat.

CONFIRMATION OF A LIPOSTAT

Two Harvard researchers, D. Mark Hegsted and Kogi Yoshinaga, and I confirmed Kennedy's results, comparing rats raised on high-fat and low-fat diets. Then we went a step further: we obtained the body composition of the rats at the time of the first estrus. After etherizing the rats, we ground up the carcasses and measured the water, protein, and fat in each rat. We found that the high-fat-diet and low-fat-diet rats indeed had the same amount of stored fat at puberty, even though the rats on the high-fat diet were younger and weighed less than the rats on the low-fat diet.

LEPTIN AS SIGNAL OF PUBERTY IN MICE — AND GIRLS

In 1997, thirty or so years after Kennedy published his results, Dr. Farid Chehab and his colleagues at the University of California, San Francisco, reported in *Science* magazine that the hormone leptin acts as a signal triggering puberty in mice. When they injected leptin into normal prepubertal female mice, the mice matured sexually much earlier than mice that had been injected with inactive salt solution. Leptin also accelerated the maturation of the tissues of the reproductive tract, the ovaries, oviducts, and uterus.

What about leptin and girls? New studies show that leptin increases in prepubertal girls, accompanying the increase in fatness that Roger Revelle and I observed during the adolescent growth spurt. Measurements of leptin in the blood of girls during the adolescent growth spurt strongly support the idea that leptin is a trigger for sexual maturation in girls as in mice.

"Neural pathways in the brain need a signal that tells them

there are enough energy stores in the body to turn on the ability to reproduce," Dr. Chehab wrote in his *Science* article. "Leptin appears to be the signal that reflects to the brain the amount of fat the individual has accumulated." Remember that growing a human infant to term requires about 50,000 calories over and above normal metabolic needs, and nursing the infant costs 500 to 1,000 calories a day. That is why storing body fat, easily mobilized energy, would have been necessary for successful reproduction in prehistoric times when the food supply was uncertain.

How might leptin signal the pubertal change? A critical concentration of leptin could activate the pulse generator of gonadotropin-releasing hormone (GnRH) in the hypothalamus. Leptin would trigger the GnRH pulse generator to produce the high-level, regular pulses which set the reproductive system on "go."

MUTANT LEPTIN GENES AND GENE RECEPTORS: NO SEXUAL DEVELOPMENT

Five unfortunate offspring of two consanguineous marriages (unions of closely related persons) provide the clinching evidence that leptin not only regulates body fat in humans but also is involved in human reproduction. One couple, married second cousins from Pakistan, carried a mutant form of the gene for leptin receptors; the other couple, from Turkey, carried a mutant form of the leptin gene itself. Because all four of these seemingly normal parents carried a hidden mutant gene, some of their offspring received two doses of the mutant gene, with disastrous results. (If only one of a pair of genes is mutant and is recessive, the normal gene of the pair dominates, functions normally, and masks the presence of the recessive mutant gene.)

The Pakistani couple carrying the mutant gene for leptin receptors had nine children, three of whom were extremely obese sisters. By analyzing the children's DNA (deoxyribonucleic acid, the fundamental chemical component of genes), investigators found that the three sisters had a homozygous mutation in the human leptin receptor gene, resulting in an abnormal leptin receptor. (A "homozygous mutation" means that both of the genes in the pair controlling the leptin receptor were abnormal.) As expected with abnormal leptin receptors, the blood of each sister had very high concentrations of leptin—twice that of the parents and of the siblings who had only one of the mutant genes.

What was unexpected was that in addition to their early onset of extreme obesity, the three unlucky sisters *had no sexual development*—no breasts, sparse pubic hair, no armpit hair, and no menstrual cycles. No sexual development also was a consequence of a mutation in the leptin gene itself.[1] Among the children of the closely related Turkish couple carrying the mutant leptin gene was an extremely obese, 22-year-old man who had two mutant versions of the leptin gene. He had low levels of leptin in his blood, as expected, but he, too, had no pubertal development. Measurement of his hormones indicated an abnormality in the signal from the hypothalamus to the pituitary gland, which normally sets the reproductive system on "go." His obese, 34-year-old sister also had two mutant leptin genes. Details of her sexual development were not known other than that she never had menstrual cycles.[2] "Life without Leptin," an article by Dr. Stephen O'Rahilly of Cambridge University, described the disastrous consequences of the mutant leptin genes. "The absolute requirement for leptin in controlling body fat mass and regulating reproduction is firmly shared between mouse and man," he observed.[3]

Another example illustrates how rapidly obesity occurs when the normal leptin gene is missing. Two cousins, a girl and a boy, were of highly consanguineous ancestry. The parents were normal themselves, but each carried a mutation in

1. K. Clément et al., "A Mutation in the Human Leptin Receptor Gene Causes Obesity and Pituitary Dysfunction," *Nature* 392 (1998): 398–401.

2. A. Strobel et al., "A Leptin Missense Mutation Associated with Hypogonadism and Morbid Obesity," *Nature Genetics* 18 (1998): 213–15.

3. Stephen O'Rahilly, "Human Physiology: Life without Leptin," *Nature* 392 (1998): 330–31.

the leptin gene. Both children gained weight very rapidly after birth, although their birth weights were normal. From early infancy on, the girl and the boy suffered from hyperphagia—they were constantly hungry, demanding food continuously, and eating much more than their normal siblings. Both children had very low levels of leptin in their blood.

By the time she was 8 years old, the girl weighed 189 pounds (86 kg); a normal 8-year-old weighs about 62 pounds (28 kg). Her 2-year-old cousin weighed 64 pounds (28 kg); normal weight for that age is about 31 pounds (14 kg). Through DNA analysis, the researchers found that both children had a homozygous mutation in the leptin gene: a single component of the normal leptin gene was missing.[4]

How leptin interacts with the human reproductive system is still being explored. It is already known that leptin is present in the fluid of the follicle, although leptin is not produced in the ovary. Also, the leptin receptor is present in the different types of ovarian cells: granulosa cells (surrounding the egg in a follicle), thecal cells (also part of a growing follicle), and interstitial cells (in the stroma of the ovary, outside the follicle). These cells secrete androgens (male hormones), which then are converted to estrogens in the ovary. Leptin apparently acts as an endocrine hormone in some way in the ovary. Thus, leptin may act on the reproductive system both at the level of the hypothalamus and pituitary and directly in the ovary, with possible implications for female reproduction, health, and disease.[5]

Leptin also has been found in the testes, in breast milk, and in the human placenta. Leptin also affects the secretion of growth hormone and thyroid hormone by the pituitary gland. More than two thousand papers have been published on leptin since its discovery; here I have presented only the major results relating to reproduction.

4. C. T. Montague et al., "Congenital Leptin Deficiency Is Associated with Severe Early-Onset Obesity in Humans," Nature 387 (1997): 903–8.

5. C. Karlsson et al., "Expression of Functional Leptin Receptors in the Human Ovary," Journal of Clinical Endocrinology and Metabolism 82, no. 12 (1997): 4144–48.

INTERACTION WITH OTHER GENES

Leptin, combined with its receptor, may also turn on other genes that affect food intake. Soon after the discovery of leptin, scientists identified a gene that functions as a short-term appetite suppressor. This regulator, called "glucagon-like factor-1," or GLP-1, acts immediately to tell the brain when it's time to stop eating. Rats that were feeding on their usual crunch food pellets suddenly stopped eating when they were injected with GLP-1.

Does GLP-1 work as an appetite suppressant in people? Scientists think it may, because GLP-1 is found in the hypothalamus of people and acts on the same systems that it controls in rats. Apparently an ancient gene, GLP-1 exists in every vertebrate species from fish to mammals. Leptin and GLP-1 may act together. When you eat a meal, your fat cells secrete leptin into the circulatory system. Leptin molecules travel to the brain and bind there to leptin receptors. The combined hormone-receptor then enters the brain cell nucleus and turns on various genes. One of the genes turned on may be an appetite suppressant like GLP-1, which is produced in the brain. When GLP-1 turns on, you stop eating because you feel full. Research on these types of interactions is proceeding apace because of the potential for new treatments for obesity and diabetes. All the drug companies are aware of the possibilities.

Many problems must be solved before leptin and GLP-1 or related substances are ready for use in humans. First, leptin must be tested for safety in animals and then, if safe for animals, it must be tested for safety in humans. Also, leptin cannot be taken orally (in a pill, for example) because it is a protein. Your digestive system would destroy it by digesting it as it does other proteins. So leptin in its present form would have to be injected, perhaps even daily. In the meantime, rely on yourself to keep your body weight in the normal range: eat a low-fat diet (not more than 30 percent of calories from fat) with lots of fruits and vegetables and exercise regularly.

LEPTIN AND BLOOD VESSELS

"Leptin initiates the growth of blood vessels." That recent finding links two of the hottest biomedical research areas, obesity and angiogenesis, the growth of new blood vessels. Yale University biochemist Dr. M. Rocío Sierra-Honigmann and her colleagues found that leptin triggers angiogenesis in experiments conducted with animals.[6]

Dr. Sierra-Honigmann made the surprising connection when she found that endothelial cells—the type of cells that form blood vessels—contain the leptin receptor. "It kept me awake at night," she reportedly said. "If I were an endothelial cell, why would I want leptin receptors?" Enlisting colleagues who study angiogenesis, she found that leptin causes endothelial cells in culture (grown in plates) to form tubes that resemble the early stages of blood vessels. Then, with the help of another researcher, they performed the "gold standard" test for whether a molecule was angiogenic: they tested whether leptin would induce new blood vessels to form in the corneas of the eyes of rats. Leptin did.

Wound healing also depends on the growth of blood vessels. Mice deficient in leptin have slower healing of wounds than normal mice. The Yale researchers have shown that extra leptin speeds healing: a normal wound in a mouse heals in five to seven days, but with leptin treatment, the wound healed completely in three to four days. In addition, slow-healing wounds of the mutant leptin-deficient mice healed like normal wounds when treated topically (on the surface) with leptin.

Leptin may be involved in the formation of new blood vessels that are needed when body fat increases. Also, because leptin is found in the fluid of follicles in the ovary, leptin may spark the growth of the numerous new blood vessels that appear when a follicle matures in the ovary in preparation for

6. M. Rocío Sierra-Honigmann et al., "Biological Action of Leptin as an Angiogenic Factor," *Science* 281 (1998): 1683–86; M. Barinaga, "Leptin Sparks Blood Vessel Growth," *Science* 281 (1998): 1582.

ovulating an egg. And, because leptin is now known to be present in the placenta, leptin may be an agent of blood vessel growth in the developing embryo.

I have been surprised by the numbers of women and men, including some medical researchers, who have never heard of leptin. I do my best to remedy the situation. Still, just to be sure my colleagues at the Population Center do not remain ignorant of this omnipresent hormone, I have hung on the wall of my office a sign sent to me by a biochemical company. It asks, "How Does Your Leptin Measure Up?" Then the uninitiated ask, "What's leptin?"

11 Population, Food Intake, and Fertility

Old and New Perspectives

I did all my research on those too lean girls and women at Harvard's Center for Population Studies. The center includes researchers from many different fields: economists and sociologists as well as demographers, who study the growth rates and changes of populations. I am the only reproductive biologist.

The only colleague to share my interest in biology was Roger Revelle, the late director of the center. Roger was an oceanographer by training, but his interests were very broad, ranging from world food supplies to growth data. We published three papers jointly on the adolescent growth spurt in girls and boys.

Roger returned from a trip to the hill country in India shortly after publication of the 1974 *Science* paper I coauthored with Janet McArthur, on fatness as a determinant of the maintenance and onset of menstrual cycles. At about the same time, the visiting economist across the hall, Warren Ilchman, who I often told about my research, asked me, "If undernutrition and intense physical activity can make women infertile, how does that apply to populations?"

I was thinking about that question when Roger, describing his trip, said to me, "Come to think of it, the women in the hill country in India are fertile only when the harvest comes in." It dawned on me then that what I had published about the later menarche of ballet dancers and athletes and the relative infertility of those lean runners and joggers might explain the lower natural fertility of couples in undernourished populations, where there was no known use of contraception, compared to noncontracepting couples in well-nourished populations like that of the United States. Living together their entire reproductive lives, the undernourished couples had six to seven children, whereas the well-nourished couples had eleven to twelve children, even though these couples married five years later than the couples with six children.

Demographers were well aware of the differences in the fertility of undernourished and well-nourished populations. Their usual explanation of the lower fertility of the undernourished populations was the use of "folk contraception." Just what was meant by "folk contraception" was not spelled out. "Folk" methods sometimes referred to withdrawal (coitus interruptus) or to customs like taboos on intercourse when women were nursing. Alternate explanations were the use of abortion or infanticide, or in some countries, venereal disease.

But, as I learned, coitus interruptus was not a widely used method of contraception in Southeast Asia, Latin America, or Africa; it was practiced mainly in continental Europe. Also, in well-studied developing countries like India, Bangladesh, and Pakistan, or among the Bush people (San) of the Kalahari desert, there was little or no evidence of abortion, infanticide, or venereal disease. Furthermore, the natural fertility of many of these populations varied from as low as four to five births per lifetime among the poorly nourished, nomadic Bush people to seven or eight births per lifetime among populations who had a good diet of coconuts and fish.

Undernutrition, Physical Work, and Female Fecundity

I proposed to my colleagues that the level of female fecundity (ability to reproduce) in a population could be adversely affected by undernutrition and strenuous physical work. A shortened reproductive life span and a lower level of reproductive efficiency, rather than folk contraception, might explain the variation in natural fertility and the smaller number of children per couple in developing countries.

You might wonder why it matters, whatever the explanation. It matters because, if I was correct, when the hoped-for improvements in socioeconomic levels of poor countries were achieved, the fertility of couples would increase—and so would the need for contraception and for the education of women to protect their reproductive health. Women would be unprepared for a rise in their ability to conceive at all ages, as I will explain.

In 1975 I was awarded a John Simon Guggenheim Memorial Foundation Fellowship to study the biological determinants of female fecundity. As soon as I began researching what nineteenth- and early twentieth-century doctors and physiologists wrote about female fecundity, I knew I was on the right track. I learned that the Northwest Indians "were only amorous when the salmon ran," and the Norwegians "had very few births when the herrings didn't run." I read these intriguing facts in the older physiological books, especially the works of the great English physiologist Francis Hugh Adam Marshall. Another Englishman, Sir Alexander Morris Carr-Saunders, studied the practices of many hunting and fishing societies and found that poor living conditions limited human ability to reproduce and better conditions enhanced it:

> Fecundity has been spoken of as if it was fixed at a certain strength for each species. As a matter of fact it varies within fairly wide limits—increasing with better conditions. In this fact lies the explanation of the increase of species under favorable conditions which has often been observed, although when conditions are less favorable, there is little or no starvation among such species.[1]

1. A. M. Carr-Saunders, *The Population Problem* (1922; New York: Arno Press, 1974), 61.

NATURE IS TELLING YOU SOMETHING

A Scottish physician, James Matthew Duncan, made the explicit connection of nutrition and fertility more than a century ago. Many medical textbooks of the time had the same theme, stating that "constitutional" reasons for sterility were more important and more prevalent than sterility caused by disease of the organs.[2] Dr. Duncan warned against being in a hurry to cure a so-called sterile woman; she may be deficient in "reproductive energy," hence if she does become pregnant, there is a high risk of miscarriage (recently confirmed), or of bearing weakly children (too lightweight—also confirmed), or of the death of the mother.[3] Another doctor, Frederick Hollick, recommended an ample diet for the sterile woman (including puddings and roast beef), as well as fresh air and sunshine, to help her "recover her flesh" and restore fertility.[4]

THE FERTILE CAREER OF THE DOMESTIC HEN

To be sure the physicians didn't miss the connection, Dr. Duncan compared the "fertile career" of women to the "fertile career of the domestic hen": the fertility of women gradually increases with age to a climax, and then gradually wanes in a manner similar to the fertile career of the domestic hen, he advised the Royal College of Physicians. Reproductive errors are more frequent at the beginning and end of the fertility curve: "An old bitch often ends her career of breeding by a dead or premature pup."[5] Dr. Duncan cited the actual number of eggs laid by a well-fed hen in its lifetime. He reported that severe underfeeding and overfeeding reduced egg-laying

2. For example, J. M. Duncan, *Fecundity, Fertility, Sterility and Allied Topics,* 2d ed. (Edinburgh: Adam and Charles Black, 1871).

3. J. M. Duncan, *On Sterility in Woman: Being the Gulstonian Lectures, Delivered in the Royal College of Physicians in February 1883* (Philadelphia: P. Blakiston, Son & Co., 1884), 113.

4. F. Hollick, *Diseases of Woman, Their Causes and Cure Familiarly Explained* (New York: T. W. Strong, 1847).

5. Duncan, *Fecundity,* p. 168.

of the hen to zero, similar to the reduction to zero of the reproductive ability of other animals, including the human female.[6]

When I plotted the number of eggs laid by Dr. Duncan's hen at different points in its lifetime, I found that the resulting curve was very similar to the age-specific fertility curve (variation of fertility with age) of women. In 1855, Dr. Duncan collected data on 16,301 married mothers from Edinburgh and Glasgow, recording the number of births per 1,000 women by age; his results appear in figure 18 below.

Dr. Duncan studied fertility by age of the mother to find the age of reproduction that was of least risk to the mother. "If a woman is to multiply and replenish the earth, as married women ordinarily do, she must survive her first confinement."[7] In 1850 and 1860 this was not an easy task: the death rate of Scottish mothers having their first child was twice as great as that of mothers during all subsequent births combined. Dr. Duncan's recommended age of 25 for marriage was based not only on mothers' survival rates but also on the late completion of the normal growth of the uterus (about age 22) and the bony pelvis (about age 25 to 30). Pelvic maturity in modern girls is still relatively late at age 21 to 24.

The doctor's interest in the changing dimensions of the pelvis with age is understandable, since fetal craniotomies—crushing the head of the fetus to remove the fetus from the uterus—were then often performed to save the life of the mother. I looked up *craniotomy* in a current obstetric text; there was no such word mentioned anywhere in it. But the nineteenth-century texts all described craniotomy as a necessary procedure in certain cases to save the life of the mother. I asked a visiting obstetrician from Egypt if he had ever heard of it and inquired why it was sometimes necessary. He explained that if a woman is undernourished or malnourished in her adolescent years, the bony pelvis can be tilted or ab-

6. Duncan, *On Sterility in Woman,* p. 113.
7. Duncan, *Fecundity,* p. 387.

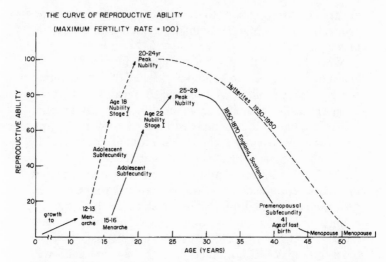

Figure 18. The curve of reproductive ability (variation of the rate of childbearing with age) among British and Scottish women in the mid-nineteenth century compared to that of well-nourished Hutterites in the mid-twentieth century. Both groups in the study married at about age 21 and did not practice contraception. The Hutterites had 11 to 12 children on average; the British and Scottish women had about 6 to 8 children. Note the earlier age of menarche and later age of menopause of the better-nourished Hutterites, who grew more rapidly and attained adult size earlier than the mid-nineteenth-century women. From R. E. Frisch, "Population, Food Intake, and Fertility," *Science* 199 (1978): 23. Reprinted with permission. Copyright © 1978 by the American Association for the Advancement of Science. Reprinted with permission of the American Association for the Advancement of Science.

normal in other ways, so a normal delivery is not possible. During the birthing process, if the mother's life is endangered and a caesarean delivery is unwise or infeasible, a craniotomy is performed and the baby removed piecemeal. "I still have to perform a craniotomy occasionally in my rural practice," he said, "but they are now rare in my city clinic." This doctor also told me that when he interned in a rural area in Maine, a frantic call came in, asking if anyone could do a craniotomy.

He was the only doctor who knew how to perform the procedure.

THE FERTILE CAREER OF
MID-NINETEENTH-CENTURY FEMALES

As my diagram above shows, the fertility career of the mid-nineteenth-century female began with menarche (or "commencing menstruation," as Dr. Duncan phrased it) at about age 15 to 16. It was already observed at that time that a period of relative infertility (now called "adolescent sterility") followed menarche. This period lasted until the completion of physical growth at about age 22, when "fitness for procreation" was attained. (Notice how late this was. American girls now finish growing at about age 16 to 18, on average.) Then came the rise to the climax, "the age of nubility," or best fitness for procreation, from age 25 to 29. This was the period of full physical vigor, when the woman had the best chance of surviving the birth of her first child.

The fertility curve then descended gradually to the age at which childbearing ceased, about 40, and then to the age at which menses ceased (menopause), about 47. Doctors had already observed that the risk of maternal mortality, infant mortality, and congenital deformities decreased from menarche to the age of nubility (25 to 29) and then increased with the advancing age of the mother.

Women in Edinburgh and Glasgow, whose fertility curve appears in figure 18 above, had about seven to eight children during their married lives. They married relatively late, about age 22 to 23, and their first child was born about seventeen months later.

Women in many developing countries at present also grow slowly to maturity and have an age-fertility curve similar to the Scottish women. Without the use of contraception, they have six to seven children in their lifetime, even though they usually marry soon after menarche. The interval from marriage to first birth can be as long as four years (as observed among the Bush people of the Kalahari desert).

THE FERTILITY CURVE
OF WELL-NOURISHED WOMEN

In contrast in the diagram above is the fertility curve of well-nourished women who do not use contraception. Well-nourished girls not only grow more rapidly to maturity, they differ in the timing of each event of the reproductive span and the level of efficiency. Menarche is earlier, adolescent sub-fecundity (often called adolescent sterility) is shorter, the age of "peak nubility" is earlier, pregnancy wastage (miscarriage and spontaneous abortion) is lower, the duration of absence of cycles (amenorrhea) with nursing is shorter, the birth interval is shorter, and the age of menopause is later and is preceded by a slower period of perimenopausal decline. The average age of menopause in the United States today is 52, compared to 45–47, historically.

Hutterite women, who do not practice contraception, have eleven or twelve births; they marry at about age 21. Their first birth is about thirteen months after marriage. Hutterite women are well nourished from birth through adulthood.

NINETEENTH-CENTURY REPRODUCTIVE TROUBLES

A look at nineteenth-century medical textbooks explains why women at that time, particularly poor women, had a shorter, less efficient reproductive life span than well-nourished women today. Back then they grew up more slowly from birth through the adolescent years because of poor diet and childhood diseases. As grown women, they continued to have a poor diet and to suffer from disease, particularly of the reproductive system. About half of all married women between the ages of 20 and 45 were reported to have "diseases of the uterus," which included amenorrhea. One-quarter of the women working in the mills suffered from either "retarded or suppressed" menses.

Amenorrhea was explained as due to "impairment of constitutional tone and impoverishment of the blood." Remedies to "bring on the changes" (menses) included hot gruel and gin to "enrich the blood and heat the system"—not a bad prescription (at least for hot gruel) in light of current knowledge. Long lists of such remedies (called emmenagogues), including drugs such as aloes, appeared in most medical books. They are distinguished from abortion-inducing drugs (called abortifacients), which apparently were little used at the time.

Doctors noted that working-class women were amenorrheic because of poor diet, disease, unsuitable employment, and cold and damp weather. Upper-class women, they reported, were amenorrheic because of their desire to be fashionably thin and also because of "violent fits of passion" (now perhaps considered stress).

Historical Linkage of Fertility and Pinguidity (Fatness)

Fatness and fertility were already specifically connected by some nineteenth-century doctors. Fatness was then referred to as "pinguidity" (from *pinguis,* the Latin word for "fat"). "She's too thin to get pregnant or to menstruate regularly" were common observations, especially when the thinness was associated with tuberculosis or with chlorosis, a virulent anemia common among working-class women that caused a sickly green color of the complexion. Dr. Hollick's prescription—giving such women puddings and roast meats and recommending fresh air and sunshine—was not a feasible one for members of the working class. "She's too fat to get pregnant" was another observation. (We know now that excessive fatness turns off menstrual cycles and ovulation.) A light diet and exercise were prescribed.

Prolapsed uterus (protrusion of the uterus through the vaginal orifice) was another common problem among women of all social classes. It could result from inadequate care at childbirth. Leukorrhea, "the whites" (a discharge from the vagina and uterus), was a standard topic in medical texts. Poor menstrual hygiene was one of the causes.

If a woman had no children by three years after marriage,

she was considered sterile. In Dr. Duncan's study of Scottish women, 15 percent of women age 15 to 44 were sterile. The level of nutrition in Scotland was not as high as in England, where the proportion of sterile women was about 10 percent. Among upper-class women, 8 percent were childless, and 7 percent had only one child. In contrast, in a well-nourished, noncontracepting modern group of women like the Hutterites, only about 2 percent are reported sterile.

NURSING AS REGULATOR OF THE BIRTH INTERVAL

In nineteenth-century England most women, including those of the upper classes, nursed their infants. It was rare to hire a wet nurse, but if a mother could not nurse, a wet nurse "who *was* and *is* well fed" was recommended.

Doctors realized then that nursing was the regulator of the birth interval. At that time, a woman who nursed had a birth interval of about two years; this interval was considered biologically natural. A two-year interval implies that a nursing mother became pregnant again at fifteen months, that is, ovulatory menstrual cycles had then resumed. But today, a well-nourished woman can nurse her infant on demand, not supplement her infant's diet, and yet have a return of a regular ovulatory cycle in as short a time as three months. (Research indicates that after six months, an infant's diet should be supplemented with more calories than can be obtained from mother's milk.) Contraception is necessary even though the mother is still nursing her infant. Otherwise, she can become pregnant and have a birth interval as short as a year. In contrast, in many developing countries, where women are not well nourished and often do physical work, the birth interval without use of contraception can be as long as thirty months.

Nineteenth-century doctors then also noticed that the length of time before the first birth after marriage also differed. Some women "low in fecundity" gave birth at greater intervals at all ages, beginning with the first birth. This variation in the ability to conceive is also found among modern women. Most of the variation is still unexplained.

DIFFERENCE IN GROWTH RATES BY SOCIAL CLASS

Girls from poor families had menarche later than girls from wealthy families, and the poor girls' physical growth and development were both later and inferior. Not surprisingly, children who worked in factories had the slowest growth, as shown in figure 19 below, and the latest sexual maturation of any of the groups studied. The factory owners had minimum standards for hiring 9-year-old girls that were amazingly low. For example, 9-year-olds had to weigh at least 48 pounds (22 kg); in 1880, English upper-class 9-year-olds weighed almost 53 pounds (24 kg). A normal 9-year-old English girl in 1965 weighed about 62 pounds (28 kg). Ironically, the standards were meant to protect the factory owners, not the children. Parents would try to palm off children who were younger than the parents said they were. Such children would faint at the looms because they didn't have the stamina and endurance to last a factory day. (Who did? one wonders: it lasted at least twelve hours.)

Measurement of adult men was popular in the 1880s. (Unfortunately, too few women were measured, so all the published data describe men.) Not only were height and weight measured for 83,000 individuals, but also chest girth, breathing capacity, and strength and span of the arms. The growth data showed that members of the well-fed and "most favored" class were taller and attained final height sooner than the ill-fed and "least favored" of the community. Most men of the lower social classes did not complete their growth in height until age 23 to 25. Even the upper-class men reached their tallest relatively late, at age 21 to 23, compared to the present age of 18 to 20 among men in the United States today.

One reason why physical growth of the social classes was so different was that what they ate was so different—a clear example of Brillat-Savarin's observation that "we are what

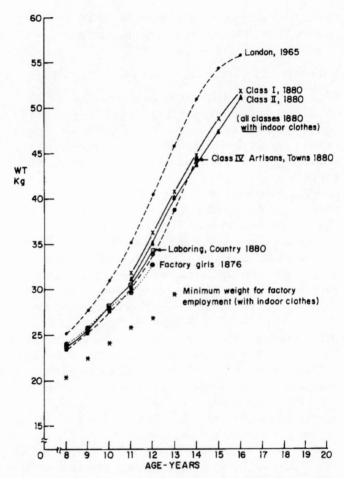

Figure 19. Body weight (kg) by age for British girls of different social classes at different times: factory girls in 1876; upper (I), middle (II to IV), and laboring/rural classes in 1880; and all girls in 1965. The minimum weights for factory employment, beginning at age 8, included clothes, as did the 1876 and 1880 weights. From R. E. Frisch, "Population, Food Intake, and Fertility," *Science* 199 (1978): 27. Copyright © 1973 by the American Association for the Advancement of Science. Reprinted with permission of the American Association for the Advancement of Science.

we eat." Wheat bread was the mainstay of the working-class diet, providing most of the calories and protein of working-class families. In very poor families, bread was almost the entire diet, supplemented with small amounts of butter, bacon, cheese, and tea. Wheat was a symbol of social status, and consumption of potatoes was at first resisted, especially by agricultural workers. After 1815, however, the price of bread rose, and potatoes became important to the working class.

Members of the middle and upper classes in Britain ate more meat and a variety of other foods, and less bread, than members of the working class. Wealthy adults and older youth ate a diet similar to that of well-off people today. A good way to find out the diet of well-off people in those days is to inquire what military officers ate. As I learned, the English officers ate well: meat, vegetables, pudding, bread, butter, milk, and beer.

DETERIORATION OF DIET
IN THE MID-NINETEENTH CENTURY

In the cities particularly, the quality of the diet among the working class deteriorated in the middle of the nineteenth century as white patent flour was substituted for whole wheat in bread, tea for ale, and jam or a little bacon for cheese. Within the family, the husband, as breadwinner, had the best diet, followed by the children and then the wife. If meat was available, most went to the husband; the wife and children ate the dripping on bread.

After 1840, sugar was cheap, and treacle (molasses) became a common spread on bread for children. Children might have bread and treacle twice a day and perhaps a boiled potato or cabbage smeared with bacon fat. The wife had mainly bread, dripping, and tea. In rural areas milk was used freely for tea, but in cities supplies were limited—a whole family's milk supply might be only one-quarter or one-half of a pint daily.

Working-class infants were often fed on "sops" (bread, water, and sugar), especially if the mother worked away from home. If a mother could not nurse and no wet nurse was available (wet nurses were unusual in England), infants were bottle fed with a siphon tube and a cow's teat. The teat was kept in gin and water, or in spirits of wine and water, so careful washing before use was recommended.

One of the reasons that working-class people fared so badly in their diet was the lack of facilities to cook hot foods. Ovens and cast-iron ranges were owned only by members of the upper classes; even cooking pots were too expensive in those times. In the country, where people kept open fires in their fireplaces, foods could be cooked if fuel was available. When fuel was too expensive or unavailable, hot meals were rare, only once or twice a week. In the cities and towns, bakers provided hot pies and tarts, in addition to bread.

In addition to the sparse diet of poor women, consider one doctor's estimates of the energy output of a worker in a spinning mill: a person attending a spinning mill walked or ran one and a third miles each hour. As mentioned earlier, a factory day was at least twelve hours, so it is not surprising that such a large proportion of the female mill workers had no menstrual cycles.

ARGUING ABOUT THE LOW FERTILITY OF THE "LOWER CLASSES"

George Udny Yule, a famous nineteenth-century economist, observed that in the 1850s, different social classes had similar fertility after marriage, about five children. Yule believed that poor people had so few children because they were undernourished and did not grow well, not because of contraception. The upper classes had so few children, he explained, because women and men married relatively late: the women after age 25, when their natural fecundity would be declining, and the men after age 30. Because the men married late, many may have frequented prostitutes, which is why many upper-class men had syphilis—a disease they gave to their wives.

Yule also observed that after about 1870, fertility began to fall in England, but the decline did not affect all classes equally: "the fall affected social strata from the top downward in rapidly decreasing degree."[8] Yule attributed the decline to the availability of an efficient contraceptive, the condom. A reliable condom was available relatively cheaply because of new processes of manufacture, especially the vulcanization of rubber. Effective female devices, diaphragms and pessaries, also became available with the advances in rubber manufacture.

But the cost of these devices in 1870 makes it improbable that they were used widely by the working class. Condoms cost two to ten shillings a dozen; rubber pessaries from two to five shillings each. There are twelve pence to the shilling, and the staple of the diet, a four-pound loaf of bread, cost about seven pence. Less effective methods were equally expensive relative to the cost of bread. The contraceptive sponge, recommended by Annie Besant, an activist for contraception for the poor, cost one shilling each. Soluble quinine pessaries cost two shillings a dozen.

A "FISH AND CHIP" BODY FAT CONNECTION?

Another and different change in England around 1870 was the increased availability of fried fish and chips as a result of the manufacture of ranges for chip frying. Growing up on fish and chips, instead of bread and dripping, would have raised the level of natural fertility considerably. Observing this, I developed a "fish and chip" hypothesis of the fall in England's birth rate: the high calorie, protein, and fat content of cheap and popular fish and chips may have increased already-improved reproductive ability among the working classes to unacceptably high levels, leading to the increased use of efficient contraception, mainly the condom, and a subsequent fall in fertility.

I first published my new perspective in a 1978 *Science* ar-

8. G. U. Yule, *The Fall of the Birth-Rate* (Cambridge: Cambridge University Press, 1920), 22.

ticle, "Population, Food Intake, and Fertility." In it I presented evidence showing how nutrition and physical work had a direct impact on fertility in a population, and the biological basis for the connection. Based on the evidence, I proposed that hoped-for improvements in economic conditions of developing countries be accompanied by an increase in family-planning programs and programs for the reproductive health of women because natural fertility would be expected to rise before it fell with the use of contraception.

With notable exceptions, my very detailed article was greeted with hostility; fortunately, the notable exceptions were demographers and economists I respected and admired. I never did understand the demographic establishment's strong opposition to this common-sense conclusion based on well-documented data. Mine wasn't even a new suggestion for a policy change. As I had mentioned in my article, C. Gopalan, director of the National Institute of Nutrition in India, published a paper six years before mine in which he stated plainly that malnourished people were less fertile than well-nourished people. When the happy time comes that everyone is well nourished, he concluded, many things will have to change, including the role of women in societies where their primary role is childbearing.

I consulted Carl Kaysen, a distinguished MIT economist then at Harvard University, to ask about one possible but unspoken reason for the demographers' opposition. If undernutrition lowered fertility, would governments of developing countries hesitate to improve diets in order to keep fertility low? "What a crazy idea!" essentially was his reply. No government could or would pursue such a policy.

FRESHENING THE COW

Perhaps the opposition of some demographers was based on ignorance of reproductive biology, as shown by the following incident. At a conference I attended on food production, an economist presented a plan for an increase in milk production. It was clear from his model that the speaker thought a cow always produced milk, just as water always come out of the tap. So as not to be confrontational, I asked, "In your scheme, how often did you plan to freshen the cow?" "Freshen the cow?" was the puzzled reply. "Well, yes, a cow gives milk only after a calf is born. Then, the milk supply gradually wanes." This was obviously a new fact to the speaker. (I even met a person from Switzerland who did not know that a cow had to have a calf to produce milk.)

But then again, maybe it wasn't lack of biological knowledge, just resistance to a new idea. I remember asking a question of a brilliant population geneticist who seemed surprised at my views. "Which do you think have more offspring, rats who spend the winter in a cold barn and eat the loose grain lying around, or the same strain of rats living in a warm basement with overflowing garbage cans?" I asked. "I don't know," replied the geneticist. This experiment was actually performed, and, of course, the warm, well-fed rats had many more little rats than the cold, lesser-fed rats: the better-fed rats began reproducing sooner, had more rats per litter, and more litters because they also kept reproducing longer.

Soon after the publication of my *Science* article, one of the notable exceptions to the adverse reaction, Professor Nathan Keyfitz of the Harvard Population Center, invited me to speak at a large international conference in Paris, honoring the memory of the Reverend Thomas Malthus. I was delighted to be in Paris, expenses paid, and glad for the opportunity to talk about my new ideas on population and environmental factors that were regarded as so unorthodox, to put it mildly, by many American demographers.

At the conference, I stood up to speak at my session at 11:30 A.M. I could see that the audience I was to address was half-asleep. There had been many speakers before me, starting at 9 A.M., and it was pleasantly warm in the hall. "What Malthus Would Have Been Surprised At" was the presentation of the previous speaker, Etienne van de Walle. Malthus was an eighteenth-century parson (sometimes called "the gloomy parson") whose famous 1798 essay on population predicted that the number of people in the world would in-

crease more rapidly than the increase in food supplies. Therefore, Malthus concluded, the death rate would rise, unless
"the preventive check of a late age of marriage was imposed"
and the further check of "moral restraint" (abstinence?)
within marriage. Professor van de Walle reassured the audience that modern agricultural technology had so far proved
Malthus wrong.

WHAT ELSE MALTHUS WOULD HAVE BEEN SURPRISED AT

To capture the attention of this somewhat soporific audience,
I began with, "Malthus would have been surprised at something else. He would have been surprised that some women
who run or jog more than twenty miles a week do not have
any menstrual cycles; they are infertile." By the time *that* was
translated into six languages, everyone in the hall was sitting
up with eyes wide open. I am sure it was the first and only oc-
casion that the phrase "menstrual cycles" echoed through
that hall in Paris.

I then presented the evidence that food intake and the
level of energy expended in physical work could explain
the observed differences of normal fertility among populations. Peter Jewell of Cambridge University and Vero Copner
Wynne-Edwards of the University of Aberdeen, who spoke
after me, described how differences in the availability of food
resulted in differences in the numbers of animal and bird
populations. The effects on humans that I had described were
consistent with their observations. The news apparently was
a surprise to the audience, who asked numerous questions.

Later, in a Left Bank restaurant, Peter Jewell and I discussed the session. Peter was an expert on the maintenance of
large-animal populations in Africa. I was enchanted to learn
from him that the age of puberty of elephants and the time
between calves of mature elephants were correlated with
changes in their environment. Peter told me that as the elephants' food supply decreased, puberty occurred later and
the interval between calves became longer, just as in girls and

women. Also, he said, elephants have menopause, and their age of menopause is also affected by the availability of food and water. When environmental conditions are good, menopause is later (the same is true for women).

A young couple was sitting at a table close to us. When I asked Peter, "Really, elephants have menopause?" the couple moved a little closer. "Oh, yes," replied Peter, "and the menopausal elephant remembers where the best watering holes are, and she leads the elephant troupe to them. So, a troupe with a menopausal elephant is healthier and has more calves than a troupe without one." By then, the neighboring couple was practically in our laps. The lady spoke: "Would you mind telling us what you two kids [*sic*] are doing in Paris?" After we explained, they told us that they were editors from an English university press, and never, in all their years in Paris, had they heard such an intriguing conversation.

My years of research on these basic connections led me to ask another controversial question: If subfecundity is the main reason for the relatively low observed fertility in the nineteenth century, who was using the many (inefficient) methods of contraception devised during human history? The likely answer was well-nourished men and women who were fully fecund and others whose reproductive capacity exceeded their aspirations for offspring. This would be a small percentage of the population: the relatively well-fed aristocracy, especially those who used wet nurses; the wet nurses themselves, because pregnancy would affect their ability to nurse; and prostitutes, whose aspirations for offspring were zero. Some demographers did not agree with my answer to this question; "folk" contraception was still supposed to have been widely used. But the evidence is otherwise, I think; why else would poor women in developing countries have so many abortions?

The nineteenth-century data raised some fundamental biological questions. The fact that undernourished human beings, as well as animals, are less fecund than those who are well nourished can be regarded as an ecological adaptation to reduced food supplies in the environment and as an obvious advantage to the population. Subfecundity is a less wasteful mechanism for the regulation of the population than is a rise in mortality.

LACK OF SAFETY OF THE RHYTHM METHOD OF CONTRACEPTION

Here is an example of how the health of women can be affected today by the lack of availability of efficient methods of contraception. Some religious groups allow only "natural" methods of contraception, namely, the rhythm method. There are two crucial times when a woman cannot safely use the rhythm method. One is when she is nursing her infant. Menstrual cycles gradually return after some months of nursing, and they may return unpredictably and irregularly. Confirming the nutrition–fertility connection, menstrual cycles and ovulation return sooner in a well-nourished woman than in a poorly nourished woman. It is very important for the health of both the mother and her infant that she not conceive again soon; if she does, her milk production will fall and her infant may fail to thrive. Also, a too close birth interval can result in a too lightweight infant. A second time a woman cannot safely use the rhythm method is around menopause, when cycles and ovulation also are irregular and when pregnancy can be dangerous for both the infant and the mother. The risk of congenital malformations such as Down's syndrome rises at this time.

And now, there is AIDS. In many countries, especially in countries of Africa and Southeast Asia, condoms are not widely available or men do not use them. Wives in villages become infected by their husbands who are returning from jobs in the cities, where they may have frequented prostitutes.

HISTORICAL DENIAL OF A WOMAN'S RIGHT TO CONTRACEPTION

The battle over a woman's right to contraception has been going on for a long time. In 1832 Dr. Charles Knowlton was sentenced to three months of hard labor in a Cambridge, Massachusetts, prison because he wrote a pamphlet telling mothers how to prevent a pregnancy, particularly while they were nursing. He recommended douching. In 1877 Annie Besant was put on trial in England with Charles Bradlaugh for republishing Dr. Knowlton's book. Trial publicity helped the book sell like hotcakes.

At the beginning of the twentieth century, and after countless prosecutions of doctors and writers who tried to help women control their fertility, Margaret Sanger had to go abroad to escape prison. She established the first clinics to help women protect themselves from too many pregnancies, which well-nourished women will have if they are not protected. In my view, it was not mere coincidence that the rise of contraceptive use and the need for its use are correlated with growing up better nourished and healthier in the United States.

A century later, politicians who understand nothing about the physiology of reproduction are still trying to prevent women and men from controlling their fertility, their reproductive health, and the health of their children. Education on the reproductive milestones of women and men and how they are affected by ordinary life circumstances, food intake, and physical activity should be part of every adolescent's curriculum—with makeup courses for adults when necessary.

Explosive Growth in World Population

Why should you care about changes in population? Because world population has exploded in size, as shown in figure 20 below. It took most of human history, up to about 1830, to populate the earth with 1 billion people, but it took only a century to double the population to 2 billion people. Forty-four years later the population doubled again, to 4 billion people, in 1975. In only twelve years another billion people were added, and by 1998 world population neared 6 billion people. There are now about 6.2 billion people in the world.

How did the population explosion happen? The difference

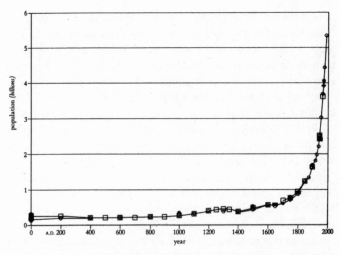

Figure 20. Estimated human population in billions from A.D. 1 to 2000. Symbols represent estimates from different sources, including the United Nations (1992). From Joel E. Cohen, *How Many People Can the Earth Support?* (New York: W. W. Norton & Co., 1995), 82. Copyright © 1995 by Joel E. Cohen. Reprinted with permission of W. W. Norton & Co., Inc.

between a population's birth rate and death rate represents the growth rate. For example, the birth rate of many developing countries is 40 births per thousand women. If the death rate is 30 per thousand people, the growth rate of the population is 1 percent, and the population doubles in about 70 years.

If the difference between the birth rate and the death rate is 2 percent (and if that seems low to you, think again), the population doubles in 35 years. At 3 percent growth, it doubles in 23 years; at 4 percent, 17.5 years. Such high growth rates are the result of decreases in death rates, made possible by the introduction of modern public health measures. Birth rates, however, remained the same until very recently, when they began falling in parts of Southeast Asia and Latin America as family planning became more widely available and women became educated about their fertility. But some African and Middle Eastern countries still have very high growth rates and therefore rapid population growth. For example, Kenya, which is relatively well off economically, has a growth rate of nearly 4 percent; it doubles its population every 18 years.

Why should these increases matter? Because the earth's capacity to support you (in the style to which you are accustomed) and the other 6 billion people on this planet is in question.

Innumerable books have been written on "the population problem," but among the most balanced is the 1995 book *How Many People Can the Earth Support?* by Joel E. Cohen, a professor at Rockefeller University. He offers "a perspective to protect you from those who say that rapid population growth is no problem at all, and from those who say that population is the only problem. A rounded view of the facts should immunize you against both cornucopians and doomsayers." Professor Cohen summarizes his view this way: "In the coming half-century, we and our children are less likely to face absolute limits than difficult tradeoffs—tradeoffs among population size and economic well-being and environmental quality and dearly held values."

The hope is that eventually, families around the world will be able to enjoy sufficient food, a good education, adequate housing, and good medical care—basically a good quality of life. But a good quality of life also includes the natural nonrenewable resources of the world, the forests, grasslands, the ocean, water in rivers and streams, and plants and animals, all of which are in danger from the rapid population growth of human beings.

12 Fatness, Fertility, and the Body Mass Index

Finding Your "Desirable Weight"

What is the desirable weight for good long-term health? What is the desirable weight to maintain fertility? How do you define being overweight or obese? These questions can be answered simply with a combined measurement called the body mass index (BMI).

"Desirable weight" is a standard adopted by researchers who gather a very large number of body weights and heights of adult women and men. These physical measurements are then evaluated in relation to the most common risk factors at older ages, such as heart disease and cancer, and also in some studies in relation to death rates.

Being overweight is defined as weighing 15–30 percent more than the desirable weight for height; being obese is defined as weighing 30 percent more than the desirable weight for height. Desirable weights for height typically have been listed in tables, like the one used by the Metropolitan Life Insurance Company.

Now the desirable, overweight, and obese weights for height are evaluated in a combined form, the BMI. The BMI conventionally uses the metric system. Your body weight is in kilograms (kg) divided by your height in meters (m) squared (multiplied by itself).

To convert to weight in pounds and height in inches, multiply your weight in pounds by 703, as shown:

$$BMI = \frac{weight \ (lb) \times 703}{height^2 \ (in)}$$

(The number 703, known as the "conversion factor," takes into account the facts that one kilogram is equal to 2.2 pounds, that there are 2.54 centimeters in one inch, and that there are 100 centimeters in one meter.)

For example, suppose a woman weighs 126 pounds (57 kg) and is 65 inches (1.65 m) tall. Her BMI is calculated as follows:

$$BMI = \frac{126 \times 703}{65 \times 65} = \frac{88,578}{4,255} = 21$$

Using the metric system directly:

$$BMI = \frac{57}{1.65 \times 1.65} = \frac{57}{2.72} = 21$$

Clinical guidelines define the desirable weight as a BMI of 20–25. Women (and men) whose BMI is 26–27 are considered moderately overweight and face moderate health risks. People with BMI over 27 are considered obese and face higher health risks.

Figure 21 below shows the BMI for individual heights and weights. Find your weight (pounds) on the scale at the left and connect it with the height (inches) closest to your own on the horizontal scale on the bottom. If you want to know your exact BMI, calculate it with the formula above using pounds and inches.

It is important to know your height precisely, not just an estimate. If you have not had your height measured recently, have it measured at your next checkup. A recent study found that adults tend to overestimate their height and underestimate their weight.

For Athletes, the BMI May Be Misleading

If you are an athlete who trains regularly, the BMI standards may not apply to you because of your increased muscle mass. (Muscles are heavier than fat: they contain 80 percent water,

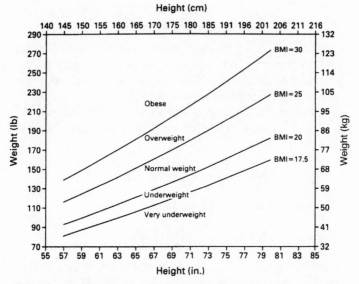

Figure 21. Body mass indexes for individual heights and weights. To chart your BMI, connect your height in inches (horizontal axis) with your weight in pounds (vertical axis), and mark the connecting point among the weight ranges (diagonal lines). Note that the body weight of athletes may not reflect their body composition because muscles are heavy (80 percent water) compared to fat (5–10 percent water). From Anne E. Becker, Steven K. Grinspoon, Anne Klibanski, and David B. Herzog, "Current Concepts: Eating Disorders," *New England Journal of Medicine* 340 (1999): 1093. Copyright © 1999 by the Massachusetts Medical Society. All rights reserved. Reprinted with permission of Anne Becker and the Massachusetts Medical Society.

whereas fat has only 5–10 percent water.) This is true especially for athletes with a BMI of 25–30. A female athlete may have the same weight as a sedentary woman of the same height but less body fat. For example, an athlete who is 65 inches tall and weighs 160 pounds has a BMI of 27. But (and it is a big "but"), direct measurements of the body fat of rowers and runners, using magnetic resonance imaging, showed that the athletes had 30–40 percent less fat than sedentary control subjects, even though their body weights were the same as or even greater than the control subjects (see chapter 9). Therefore, the BMI of women who exercise regularly may be misleading because their body weight has a higher proportion of muscle.

Weight remains relatively stable for young women up to age 25 to 30. Then weight begins to increase mainly from an increase in body fat (as you can see in figure 7, chapter 6). For long-term health, the recommendation is to keep your weight in the normal range of BMI, 20–25, with a low-fat diet and regular exercise.

FERTILITY AND YOUR BMI

A BMI in the range of 20 to 25 is associated with normal fertility.

On the Underweight Side

Remember that in order to maintain normal ovulatory menstrual cycles and to become pregnant, you must not be too thin or too lean; see chapters 6 and 7.

The "minimum" weight for a particular height for maintenance of normal ovulatory cycles, which I describe in chapter 6, is equivalent to a BMI of 18. For example, for a height of 65 inches, the minimum weight is 108 pounds. If you want to become pregnant, it is advisable to have a BMI above 18.

$$BMI = \frac{108 \times 703}{65 \times 65} = \frac{75,924}{4,255} = 18$$

Research indicates that the hormonal environment for a successful pregnancy outcome will be improved with a BMI over 19.

On the Overweight Side

A BMI of 25–27 is associated with a slight reduction in fertility; over 27 with a significantly reduced fertility.

In summary, for good health and normal fertility, keep your BMI in the range of 20 to 25.[1]

1. R. L. Barbieri, A. D. Domar, and K. R. Loughlin, *Six Steps to Increased Fertility* (New York: Simon and Schuster, 2000).

BIOGRAPHICAL NOTE

If the scientific saga I have recounted seems unusual, that is because it *was* unusual.

When I returned to work after my children were grown, I had already earned my doctoral degree in genetics; my thesis, luckily for my later research, was on growth rates. But genetics had become molecular, and I wanted to work on a broader current problem like population growth. So I applied to the newly opened Harvard Center for Population Studies, part of the Harvard School of Public Health.

The center hired me as a research assistant for four dollars an hour to work on the World Food Needs Project. I was glad to get my foot in the door, and I figured there was nowhere to go but up. I probably got the job because I had recently published a successful book, *Plants That Feed the World,* which I had written at Harvard's fine economic botany library. Now, thirty years later, I am a professor emerita at Harvard's School of Public Health—and in those intervening years, I did the research described in this book.

Research on new ideas is not often funded by the national agencies, foundations, and other powers that dispense money. But I was fortunate that when I began work at my lowly salary, I did not need to support myself or my early research on body fat and fertility. My husband was a professor of physics at the Massachusetts Institute of Technology, so that took care of finances. I could use my Harvard salary for stamps.

In 1975, when I began teaching my own graduate course on female fertility, the center provided me with a research assistant and increased my salary slightly. By then I was a lecturer, a nonprofessorial slot typical for women teaching in

176   BIOGRAPHICAL NOTE

the medical area at the time. (In those days, it was very hard
to climb out of that slot.) When I was awarded a John Simon
Guggenheim Memorial Foundation fellowship in 1975, the
foundation asked me for my salary. When I wrote them the
amount, they called me up and said, "Not your monthly
salary, your *annual* salary." "That *is* my annual salary," I
replied. The center then gave me a raise.

But I was very fortunate because I could follow any clues I
pleased. Roger Revelle provided intellectual support, as did
interested physicians at Harvard Medical School with whom
I collaborated. Very important, I had access to all the Harvard libraries, including the Countway Library of Medicine.
Later I received financial support for my research from the
National Institutes of Health, the Advanced Medical Research Foundation, and the National Science Foundation.

I am still doing research on the reproductive health of
adolescent girls and women in relation to the body fat connection.

GLOSSARY

ADIPOCYTES. Fat cells.

ADIPOSE TISSUE. Body fat, consisting of the fat cell (the *adipocyte*) and connective tissue (the *stroma*).

AMENORRHEA. The absence of menstrual cycles, causing infertility.

AMPULLA. The enlarged, middle part of the fallopian tube where the egg awaits fertilization by the sperm.

ANDROGENS. Steroid hormones secreted by the testis and the adrenal glands.

ANOVULATORY. The absence of ovulation in a menstrual cycle, causing infertility.

ENDOMETRIUM. The lining of the uterus.

ESTROGEN. A steroid hormone, secreted by the ovaries, that regulates the development of the uterus, the breasts, and other tissues of the female reproductive tract. Estrogen also regulates the characteristic deposition of female fat in the hips, thighs, and breasts.

ESTRUS. Sexual maturation in nonprimate mammals. The *estrous period* is a phase of sexual receptivity known popularly as being "in heat."

FECUNDITY. Reproductive ability.

FOLLICULAR PHASE. The phase of the menstrual cycle up to ovulation characterized by growth of an ovarian follicle, which contains an egg (the *ovum*), and rapid growth of the lining of the uterus (*endometrium*). This period normally lasts about fourteen days.

FOLLICLE-STIMULATING HORMONE (FSH). A hormone secreted by the pituitary gland that promotes the growth of the ovum and ovarian follicles.

GAMETES. Egg and sperm cells. Gametes have 23 chromosomes, half the number of somatic (body) cells.

GONADOTROPIN-RELEASING HORMONE (GnRH). A hormone secreted by the hypothalamus that controls the release of follicle-stimulating hormone (FSH) and luteinizing hormone (LH) by the pituitary gland.

HYPOTHALAMUS. Part of the third ventricle of the brain (the *diencephalon*) that controls the ability to reproduce in addition to food and water intake, energy metabolism, sleep, body temperature, and emotions. Among other functions, the hypothalamus secretes releasing hormones that control the cascade of pituitary hormones, which in turn control the reproductive system.

LACTATION. The secretion of milk in the breast; breast feeding.

LEPTIN. A protein hormone made by fat cells that reduces appetite and increases energy metabolism. Leptin is now regarded as one of the protein hormones that keeps body weight in the normal range over long periods. Receptors for leptin are located in the hypothalamus. Leptin is involved in reproduction.

LUTEINIZING HORMONE (LH). A hormone secreted by the pituitary gland that, together with follicle-stimulating hormone, stimulates estrogen secretion. The surge of LH in the middle of the menstrual cycle stimulates ovulation. LH then controls the transformation of the ruptured ovarian follicle to become the *corpus luteum* ("yellow body"), which secretes both estrogen and progesterone.

LUTEAL PHASE. The period of the menstrual cycle after ovulation during which the uterine lining (*endometrium*) prepares for implantation of the fertilized egg. If this does not occur, the uterus sheds its lining and menstruation occurs, normally about fourteen days after ovulation.

MENARCHE. The first menstrual cycle. This cycle can often be without ovulation, and the following menstrual cycles may be irregular for one or two years.

OVULATION. The release of the egg from the ovary, usually occurring fourteen days after menstruation.

PITUITARY GLAND. The "master" endocrine gland, it is controlled by the relasing factors of the hypothalamus and regulates the other endocrine organs of the body, including the ovary and testis. The hypothalamus triggers the pituitary gland to secrete two principal hormones necessary for ovulation, follicle-stimulating hormone (FSH) and luteinizing hormone (LH).

PUBERTY. A general term covering the period of time of the adolescent growth spurt and the development of secondary sex characteristics such as breast development and pubic hair in girls; it precedes menarche. (Some doctors include menarche.)

SUBFECUNDITY. A low ability to reproduce.

TESTOSTERONE. An androgen produced by the testis. Testosterone regulates the development of genitalia and characteristics of the skeleton and muscular system in men.

SUGGESTIONS FOR
FURTHER READING

CLASSICS

Carr-Saunders, A. M. *The Population Problem*. 1922. Reprint, New York: Arno Press, 1974.

Corner, G. W. *The Hormones in Human Reproduction*. Princeton: Princeton University Press, 1946.

Corner, G. W. *Anatomist at Large*. New York: Basic Books, 1958.

Duncan, J. M. *Fecundity, Fertility, Sterility, and Allied Topics*. 2d ed., rev. and enl. Edinburgh: Adam and Charles Black, 1871.

Hammond, John. *Farm Animals: Their Breeding, Growth, and Inheritance*. London: Edward Arnold & Co., 1940.

Marshall, F. H. A. *The Physiology of Reproduction*. 2d ed. London: Longmans Green, 1922.

Moore, F. K., H. Oleson, J. D. McMurrey, V. Parker, M. R. Ball, and L. M. Boyden. *The Body Cell Mass and Its Supporting Environment*. Philadelphia: W. B. Saunders Co., 1963.

Quetelet, Adolphe. *A Treatise on Man and the Development of His Faculties*. 1842. Trans. R. Knox and T. Smibert. Reprint, New York: Burt Franklin, 1968.

Renold, A. E., and G. F. Cahill Jr., eds. *Adipose Tissue*. Handbook of Physiology, Section 5. Washington, D.C.: American Physiological Society, 1965.

MORE RECENT BOOKS

Barbieri, R. L., A. D. Domar, and K. R. Loughlin, *Six Steps to Increased Fertility* (New York: Simon and Schuster, 2000).

Cohen, J. E. *How Many People Can the Earth Support?* New York: W. W. Norton and Co., 1995.

Frisch, R. E., ed. *Adipose Tissue and Reproduction*. Basel, Switzerland: Karger, 1990.

Fryer, Peter. *The Birth Controllers*. New York: Stein and Day, 1965.

McClung, Jean. *Effects of High Altitude on Human Birth*. Cambridge: Harvard University Press, 1969.

ARTICLES AND ESSAYS

Apter, D., N. J. Bolton, G. L. Hammond, and R. Vihko. "Serum Sex Hormone-Binding Globulin during Puberty in Girls and in Different Types of Adolescent Menstrual Cycles." *ACTA Endocrinologica* 107 (1984): 413–19.

Bernstein, L., B. E. Henderson, R. Hanish, J. Sullivan-Halley, and R. H. Ross. "Physical Exercise and Reduced Risk of Breast Cancer in Young Women." *Journal of the National Cancer Institute* 86 (1994): 1403–8.

Boyar, R. M., J. Katz, J. W. Finkelstein, S. Kapen, H. Weiner, E. D. Weitzman, and L. Hellman. "Anorexia Nervosa: Immaturity of the 24-hour Luteinizing Hormone Secretory Pattern." *New England Journal of Medicine* 291 (1974): 861–65.

Eastman, N. J., and E. Jackson. "Weight Relationships in Pregnancy. I: The Bearing of Maternal Weight Gain and Pre-pregnancy Weight on Birth Weight in Full Term Pregnancies." *Obstetrical and Gynecological Survey* 23 (1968): 1003–25.

Edelman, I. S., H. B. Haley, P. R. Schloerb, D. B. Sheldon, B. J. Friis-Hansen, G. Stoll, and F. D. Moore. "Further Observations on Total Body Water. I. Normal Values throughout the Life Span." *Surgery, Gynecology and Obstetrics* 95 (1952): 1–12.

Emerson, K., Jr., B. N. Saxena, and E. L. Poindexter. "Caloric Cost of Normal Pregnancy." *Obstetrics and Gynecology* 40 (1972): 786–94.

Friis-Hansen, B. "Changes in Body Water Compartments during Growth." *Acta Paeditrica Scandinavia,* supp. 110 (1956): 1–67.

Frisch, R. E. "Demographic Implication of the Biological Determinants of Female Fecundity." *Social Biology* 22 (1975): 17–22.

———. "Fatness of Girls from Menarche to Age 18 Years, with a Nomogram." Human Biology 48 (1976): 353–59.

———. "Population, Food Intake, and Fertility: Historical Evidence for Direct Effect of Nutrition on Reproductive Ability." *Science* 199 (1978): 2–30.

———. "Fatness, Puberty, and Fertility." *Natural History* 89 (1980): 16–27. Reprinted in *Introduction to Human Ecology,* ed. G. F. Clark. Dubuque, Iowa: Kendall/Hunt Publishing Co., 2000.

———. "Pubertal Adipose Tissue: Is It Necessary for Normal Sexual Maturation? Evidence from the Rat and the Human Female." Federation Proceedings 39 (1980): 2395–400.

———. "What's Below the Surface?" New England Journal of Medicine 305 (1981): 1019–20 (correspondence).

———. "Fatness, Menarche, and Female Fertility." Perspectives in Biology and Medicine 28 (1985): 611–33.

———. "Maternal Nutrition and Lactational Amenorrhea: Perceiving the Metabolic Cost." In Maternal Nutrition and Lactational Infertility, ed. J. Dobbing, 65–91. New York: Raven Press, 1985.

———. "Fatness and Fertility." Scientific American 258 (1988): 88–95.

———. "Body Fat, Menarche, Fitness, and Fertility." In Adipose Tissue and Reproduction, ed. R. E. Frisch, 1–26. Basel, Switzerland: Karger, 1990.

Frisch, R. E., D. M. Hegsted, and K. Yoshinaga. "Body Weight and Food Intake at Early Estrus of Rats on a High Fat Diet." Proceedings of the National Academy of Science (USA) 72 (1975): 4172–76.

———. "Carcass Components at First Estrus of Rats on High Fat and Low Fat Diets: Body Water, Protein, and Fat." Proceedings of the National Academy of Science 74 (1977): 379–83.

Frisch, R. E., J. A. Canick, and D. Tulchinsky. "Human Fatty Marrow Aromatizes Androgen to Estrogen." Journal of Clinical Endocrinology and Metabolism 51 (1980): 394–96.

Frisch, R. E., G. M. Hall, T. T. Aoki, J. Birnholz, R. Jacob, L. Landsberg, H. Munro, K. Parker-Jones, D. Tulchinsky, and J. Young. "Metabolic, Endocrine, and Reproductive Changes of a Woman Channel Swimmer." Metabolism: Clinical and Experimental 33 (1984): 1106–11.

Frisch, R. E., and J. W. McArthur. "Menstrual Cycles: Fatness as a Determinant of Minimum Weight for Height Necessary for Their Maintenance or Onset." Science 185 (1974): 949–51.

Frisch, R. E., R. C. Snow, L. A. Johnson, B. Gerard, R. L. Barbieri, and B. Rosen. "Magnetic Resonance Imaging of Overall and Regional Body Fat, Estrogen Metabolism, and Ovulation of Athletes Compared to Controls." Journal of Clinical Endocrinology and Metabolism 77 (1993): 471–77.

Frisch, R. E., A. von Gotz-Welbergen, J. W. McArthur, T. Albright, J. Witschi, B. Bullen, J. Birnholz, R. B. Reed, and H. Hermann. "Delayed Menarche and Amenorrhea of College Athletes in Relation to Age of Onset of Training." *Journal of the American Medical Association* 246 (1981): 1559–63.

Frisch, R. E., G. Wyshak, N. Albright, T. Albright, I. Schiff, K. Parker-Jones, J. Witschi, E. Shiang, E. Koff, and M. Marguglio. "Lower Prevalence of Breast Cancer and Cancers of the Reproductive System among Former College Athletes Compared to Non-Athletes." *British Journal of Cancer* 52 (1985): 885–91.

Frisch, R. E., G. Wyshak, T. Albright, and I. Schiff. "Lower Prevalence of Diabetes in Female Former College Athletes Compared with Non-Athletes." *Diabetes* 35 (1986): 1101–5.

Frisch, R. E., G. Wyshak, and L. Vincent. "Delayed Menarche and Amenorrhea in Ballet Dancers." *New England Journal of Medicine* 303 (1980) 17–19.

Hileman, S. M., D. D. Perroz, and J. S. Flier. "Leptin, Nutrition, and Reproduction: Timing Is Everything." *Journal of Clinical Endocrinology and Metabolism* 85 (2000): 804–7.

Hill, J. O., and J. C. Peters. "Environmental Contributions to the Obesity Epidemic." *Science* 280 (1998): 1371–74.

Kennedy, G. C. "Interactions between Feeding Behavior and Hormones during Growth." *Annals of the New York Academy of Science* 157 (1969): 1049–61.

Kennedy, G. C., and J. Mitra. "Body Weight and Food Intake as Initiation Factors for Puberty in the Rat." *Journal of Physiology* 166 (1963): 408–18.

Marshall, F. H. A., and W. R. Peel. "'Fatness' as a Cause of Sterility." *Journal of Agricultural Science* 3 (1908): 383–89.

Mellits, E. D., and D. Cheek. "The Assessment of Body Water and Fatness from Infancy to Adulthood." In *Physical Growth and Body Composition*, ed. J. Brožek, 12–26. Monographs of the Society for Research in Child Development, vol. 35, no. 7. Chicago: University of Chicago Press, 1970.

Nimrod, A., and K. J. Ryan. "Aromatization of Androgens by Human Abdominal and Breast Fat Tissue." *Journal of Clinical Endocrinology and Metabolism* 40 (1975): 367–72.

Sargent, D. W. "Weight–Height Relationship of Young Men and Women." *American Journal of Clinical Nutrition* 13 (1963): 318–25.

Scammon, R. E. "The Measurement of the Body in Childhood." In *The Measurement of Man,* ed. A. J. Harris, C. M. Jackson, and D. G. Paterson, 174–215. Minneapolis: University of Minnesota Press, 1930.

Vague, J., and R. Fenasse. "Comparative Anatomy of Adipose Tissue." In *Adipose Tissue,* Handbook of Physiology, Section 5, ed. A. E. Renold and G. F. Cahill Jr., 25–26. Washington, D.C.: American Physiological Society, 1965.

Vigersky, R. A., A. E. Andersen, R. H. Thompson, and D. L. Loriaux. "Hypothalamic Dysfunction in Secondary Amenorrhea Associated with Simple Weight Loss." *New England Journal of Medicine* 297 (1977): 1141–45.

Warren, M. P., R. Jewelewicz, I. Dyrenfurth, R. Ans, S. Khalaf, and R. L. Vande Weile. "The Significance of Weight Loss in the Evaluation of Pituitary Response to LH–RH in Women with Secondary Amenorrhea." *Journal of Clinical Endocrinology and Metabolism* 40 (1975): 601–11.

"Weight and Longevity." *Harvard Health Letter* 23, no. 5 (1998).

Widdowson, E. M. "Biological Implications of Body Composition." In *Body Composition in Animals and Man.* Publication 1598, National Academy of Sciences, Washington, D.C., 1968.

Wyshak, G., and R. E. Frisch. "Evidence for a Secular Trend in Age of Menarche." *New England Journal of Medicine* 306 (1982): 1033–35.

INDEX

Abortifacients, 155
Adipocytes, 5, 6
Adipose body, 20, 21
Adipose tissue. *See* Body fat
Adipose Tissue and Reproduction
(Frisch, ed.), 90–92
Adolescence, female, 22–37; adolescent growth spurt, 22–23, 24–27, 48, 65–66, 71; bone mass formation, 134; changes in body composition, 66–67; peak weight gain, 23–24. *See also* Menarche
Adolescence, male, 36–37
Adolescent sterility, 153
Adrenal cortex, 7
Adrenal gland, 6
Adrostenedione, 7
Aging, water content and, 67
AIDS, 166
Albright, Hollis, 97
Albright, Nile, 97
Albright, Tenley, 97, 116
Allen, Willard, 91–92
Altitude, high: and birth weight, 32; and delay of menarche, 31–33
Alumnae Health Study, 113–36; athlete characteristics, 116–17; body fat measurement using MRI, 123–26; collecting family and medical histories, 114–16; findings regarding bone fractures, 130–31; findings regarding breast cancer and reproductive-system cancers, 117–20, 121–23; findings regarding consump-

tion of cola, 131–35; findings regarding late-onset diabetes, 128–30; findings regarding nonpotent estrogen, 126–27; findings regarding other types of cancers, 127–28; follow up, 135–36
Amenorrhea, 8, 17, 48; in nineteenth century, 154–55, 160; primary and secondary, 97
Amino acids, 48
Ampulla, 45, 51
Androgens, 7, 85, 122, 143
Angiogenesis, 85, 145–46
Animals: fat and reproduction in, 13, 20–21; mammals' body composition, 12–13
Anorexia nervosa, 14, 48, 101; predicting menarche for girls with, 72–74; recovery from, illustrated, 77
Anovulatory menstrual cycles, 54
Aphrodite of Kyrene, 123, 125
Apocrine sweat, 36–37
Appetite suppressant, leptin and, 144
Apter, Dan, 122
Aromatase, 7, 85
Aromatization, 7–8
Athletes: and body mass index, 171–73; delayed menarche, 99–101; differences from anorectics, 101; differences in pre- and postmenarcheal, 100; effect of low percentage of body fat on menstrual cycles, 12, 80; food